KU-279-705

MRCS

Volume 1

Core Modules

Commissioning Editor: Laurence Hunter
Project Development Manager: Barbara Simmons
Project Controller: Frances Affleck
Designer: Judith Wright

The Complete
MRCS
Volume 1
Core Modules

Edited by

Joseph K. C. Huang FRCS
Specialist Registrar in General Surgery
Anglia/Cambridge Region

Marc C. Winslet MS FRCS
Professor of Surgery and Head of Department
Royal Free Hospital and
University College Medical School
London

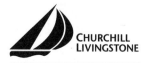
CHURCHILL
LIVINGSTONE

EDINBURGH   LONDON   NEW YORK   PHILADELPHIA   ST LOUIS   SYDNEY   TORONTO   2000

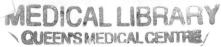
CHURCHILL LIVINGSTONE
An imprint of Harcourt Publishers Limited

© Harcourt Publishers Limited 2000

 is a registered trademark of Harcourt Publishers Limited

First published 2000

ISBN 0443 06458X

British Library Cataloguing in Publication Data
A catalogue record for this book is available from the British Library

Library of Congress Cataloging in Publication Data
A catalog record for this book is available from the Library of Congress

Medical knowledge is constantly changing. As new information becomes available, changes in treatment, procedures, equipment and the use of drugs become necessary. The editors and the publishers have, as far as it is possible, taken care to ensure that the information given in this text is accurate and up to date. However, readers are strongly advised to confirm that the information, especially with regard to drug usage, complies with the latest legislation and standards of practice.

The
publisher's
policy is to use
**paper manufactured
from sustainable forests**

Printed by Bell & Bain Ltd., Glasgow

Preface

The aim of this book is to assist candidates in their final preparation for the MRCS examination, by allowing self-assessment of major parts of the syllabus, which will highlight areas of deficiency. It is not intended to be a comprehensive overview of the syllabus, which is already provided in the distance learning or STEP course published by the Royal College of Surgeons of England.

By their nature books containing MCQs cover certain areas in greater depth than others. It is not intended that the text should represent a substitute for extensive clinical reading, but rather act as a complement to it.

Each question includes a short answer section containing relevant background information and clinical comment where appropriate. Some of the answers will generate discussion and controversy reflecting normal clinical practice and hopefully stimulating further research and evaluation.

London, 2000

M. C. W.
J. K. C. H.

Contributors

Ragheed A. M. Al-Mufti MB MSC
MD FRCS (Gen)
Consultant Surgeon,
Whittington Hospital, London
Questions and answers 1.1–1.53

Tim Davidson ChM MRCP FRCS
Consultant Surgeon,
Royal Free Hospital, London
Questions and answers 5.34–5.66

Adrian Fogarty FRCS FRCSED(A&E)
FFAEM
Consultant in Accident
and Emergency Medicine,
Royal Free Hospital, London
Questions and answers 3.1–3.36

Emma Gray MS FRCS
Specialist Registrar in General
Surgery, North-East Thames
Region, London
Questions and answers 5.1–5.33

Stephen Hallworth FRCA
Research Fellow in Anaesthesia,
Royal Free Hospital, London
Questions and answers 4.1–4.51

Joseph K. C. Huang FRCS
Specialist Registrar in General
Surgery, Anglia/Cambridge
Region
Questions and answers 5.67–5.76

Tim Issitt FRCA
Specialist Registrar in
Anaesthesia, North-East Thames
Region, London
Questions and answers 4.1–4.51

Bryony Lovett MChir FRCS (Gen)
Lecturer in Surgery, University
College Hospital, London
Questions and answers 2.1–2.33

Larry Mulleague FRCA
Specialist Registrar in
Anaesthesia, North-East Thames
Region, London
Questions and answers 4.1–4.51

S. A. Wajed FRCS
Specialist Registrar, North-East
Thames Region, London;
Research Fellow, Department
of Surgery, University of Southern
California, USA
Questions and answers 5.44–5.76

Marc C. Winslet MS FRCS
Professor of Surgery and Head
of Department, Royal Free
Hospital and University College
Medical School, London
Questions and answers 2.1–2.33
Questions and answers 5.34–5.43

Contents

Questions

Core module 1
Perioperative management (I)   1

Core module 2
Perioperative management (II)   17

Core module 3
Trauma   27

Core module 4
Intensive care   39

Core module 5
Neoplasia, the breast, and
techniques and outcome of surgery   53

Answers

Core module 1
Perioperative management (I)   75

Core module 2
Perioperative management (II)   99

Core module 3
Trauma   113

Core module 4
Intensive care   137

Core module 5
Neoplasia, the breast, and
techniques and outcome of surgery   165

Index   199

CORE MODULE **1**

Perioperative management (I)

1.1 Wound healing by secondary intention takes place:
A. When the wound does not break apart.
B. When the wound edges are brought together.
C. When there is irreparable skin loss.
D. Much more slowly than healing by first intention.
E. When the wound becomes infected.

1.2 Acute metabolic acidosis in emergency surgery:
A. Does not occur in the total body hypoxia seen in cardiac arrest.
B. Is the result of inadequate tissue perfusion.
C. Is related to the activation of aerobic pathways of energy supply.
D. Is associated with prolonged cross-clamping of the aorta during aneurysm repair.
E. Is present when the whole body has been underperfused for an hour.

1.3 Early septic shock postoperatively:
A. Does not require early dialysis, if there is a rapid rise in serum creatinine and urea.
B. Presents with warm hypotension which may progress to cold hypotension with reduced cardiac output and high peripheral vascular resistance.
C. Is associated with a low mortality if it presents with 'cold hypotension'.
D. Is part of the systemic immune response syndrome.
E. Is often of the hyperdynamic type.

1.4 **In preventing infection at operation:**
  A. The open wound is at risk of contamination from airborne dust, and bacteria from skin organisms of operating room personnel.
  B. Positive pressure filtered ventilation of the operating theatre does not prevent bacteria gaining entry with the air.
  C. Ultra-clean ventilation with laminar flow and fine filter reduces the rate of wound infection tenfold.
  D. The patient's own skin is not a source of infection especially in abdominal operations.
  E. The use of a plastic adhesive film (Opsite), through which the incision is made, prevents contamination.

1.5 **The following statements concerning necrotizing fasciitis are correct:**
  A. Antibiotic therapy and hyperbaric oxygen do not limit the spread.
  B. There is a severe infective process, but the skin initially appears normal.
  C. Conservative excision of the necrotic fascia and skin and muscle should be carried out within 24 h.
  D. It is not common after minor trauma or in intravenous drug abusers.
  E. High doses of benzylpenicillin (4 mega units) given intravenously are indicated.

1.6 **Early wound infection and inflammation are characterized by:**
  A. Decreased blood flow.
  B. Increased vascular permeability.
  C. Local infiltration of cells that phagocytose microbes and damaged tissue.
  D. Association with a deep-seated abscess collection.
  E. An inflammatory response which is dependent on the burden of tissue injury.

1.7 **In the management of surgical wound infections:**
  A. Surgical debridement of damaged tissue is not essential.
  B. Excess retraction of small wounds does not affect the infection rate.
  C. Complete haemostasis is essential.
  D. The presence of a deadspace during wound closure does not delay wound healing.
  E. The wound should be closed with layer-to-layer approximation without tension.

1.8 **A prolonged period of therapy with parenteral antibiotics is indicated:**
  A. When there is progression of infection despite adequate drainage.
  B. In immunocompromised patients.
  C. For the treatment of uncomplicated wound abscesses which can be drained surgically.
  D. When there is evidence of septicaemia.
  E. For anaerobic cover in colonic surgery.

1.9 **Factors that increase the risk of surgical patients acquiring infection include:**
  A. Hypoalbuminaemia.
  B. Morbid obesity.
  C. Concurrent sepsis.
  D. The location and duration of operation.
  E. Long-term use of prophylactic antibiotics.

1.10 **Factors that reduce the risk of abdominal wound dehiscence include:**
  A. Mass muscle closure with interrupted absorbable or polymer sutures.
  B. Wound healing by secondary intention in the presence of major intra-abdominal sepsis.
  C. Closure with continuous suture, the length of its material being twice as long as the surgical incision.
  D. Reducing the risk of wound infection with antibiotic prophylaxis at induction.
  E. Preoperative TPN to correct malnutrition.

‣1.11 Wound healing can be improved by:
  A. Meticulous surgical technique and avoiding wound infection.
  B. Skin shaving 24–48 h before surgery.
  C. Incising the skin along the lines of Langer.
  D. Local injection of steroids.
  E. Use of prophylactic antibiotics for five days postoperatively.

1.12 The APACHE II scoring system for preoperative assessment:
  A. Is the system used by the Surgical Infection Society to compare treatment regimens.
  B. Uses disease-specific weighting factors to calculate morbidity.
  C. Does not depend on the Glasgow Coma Scale for its evaluation.
  D. Is greatly affected by chronic conditions affecting the liver, cardiovascular and pulmonary function. These affect both the APACHE II score and the mortality risk.
  E. Correlates with a mortality risk of 50% if there is a score above 21.
  F. Consists of an acute physiology score and a chronic health evaluation.

‣ 1.13 Adverse effects of perioperative blood transfusion include:
  A. Cytomegalovirus (CMV) infection.
  B. Iron overload.
  C. Alloimmunization.
  D. Transfusion-associated host-versus-graft disease.
  E. Hepatitis B and C infections.

1.14 In synergistic gangrene:
  A. The initial cellulitis is followed by progressive gangrenous ulceration.
  B. Chronic progressive bacterial gangrene is caused by the synergistic action of aerobic haemolytic Staphylococci and microaerophilic non-haemolytic Streptococci.
  C. Meleney's burrowing ulcers are caused by Staphylococci alone.
  D. The skin necrosis is characterized by a metallic sheen.
  E. All Clostridia (in gas gangrene) owe their pathogenicity to elaboration of soluble endotoxins that destroy tissue and blood cells.
  F. The diagnosis of gas gangrene is based on typical clinical findings, as well as on the presence of large Gram-positive rods in the wound fluid.

1.15 In cases of surgical infection:
  A. Contamination of the abdominal cavity can only follow penetrating abdominal trauma.
  B. Secondary peritonitis in traumatic intestinal rupture is a common feature when the patient undergoes a laparotomy after 24 h.
  C. Curtis–Fitz–Hugh syndrome may mimic cholecystitis, and can be treated with antibiotics.
  D. Obligate anaerobes are commonly found in liver abscesses.
  E. A localized paracolic diverticular abscess can be drained percutaneously under ultrasound or CT guidance.
  F. Pancreatitis begins as an infection but most of the fatalities are caused by a chemical inflammation.

1.16 In cases of postoperative wound infection:
  A. Reopening the wound and evacuating the pus is the optimal treatment for infections with a collection.
  B. Diagnosis depends on the results of a gram stain of needle-aspirated material, irrespective of the clinical findings.
  C. Rate is increased in proportion to the time elapsed between skin shaving and operation.
  D. Antibiotic prophylaxis is effective in preventing postoperative infection when given 3 h following surgery.
  E. The earliest sign of superficial infection is local erythema without pain or induration.
  F. The infection is independent of the nutritional status of the patient.

1.17 The following statements are true:
  A. Adequate laminar flow system in the operating theatres is not essential in order to perform sterile surgical procedures.
  B. Interrupted vertical mattress sutures are used where the skin edges may not approximate accurately because of tissue laxity.
  C. Modern electrocautery machines employ a rheostat to vary the output current to achieve haemostasis.
  D. The bipolar diathermy machine uses a low current at very high frequency and high voltage, which is passed through the patient's tissue using two electrodes to complete the circuit.
  E. Bipolar diathermy should be used if the patient has a pacemaker in place.

1.18 Preoperative chest X-ray is required in:
  A. A patient with chronic respiratory symptoms, although with normal chest X-ray six months earlier.
  B. A patient with cardiomyopathy with normal chest X-ray six months earlier.
  C. A 50-year-old patient undergoing routine abdominal operation.
  D. A 30-year-old patient with malignancy.
  E. A 25-year-old patient who is a recent immigrant.

1.19 Heparin anticoagulation:
A. Is reversed by the administration of Vitamin K.
B. Has longer action when administered intravenously than subcutaneously.
C. Side effects include thrombocytopenia.
D. Is cleared from the body mainly by renal excretion.
E. Can be used subcutaneously to treat iliac vein thrombosis by twice daily administration of low molecular weight heparin.

1.20 Appropriate investigations for staging a 70-year-old male smoker prior to total gastrectomy for malignancy include the following:
A. Liver function test.
B. Chest X-ray.
C. Laparoscopy.
D. Barium swallow.
E. Gastroscopy.

1.21 These problems are associated with morbid obesity in patients undergoing abdominal surgery:
A. Deep venous thrombosis occurs infrequently preoperatively.
B. Laparoscopic surgery is often easier for patients and surgeons.
C. There is an increased tendency to hypertension, diabetes and arthritis.
D. There is an increased incidence of wound haematoma.
E. Wound infection and dehiscence are more likely.

1.22 The following statements are true of thyroid cancer:
A. Should be treated by subtotal thyroidectomy in papillary carcinoma.
B. ^{131}I therapy has no role to play in the preoperative management.
C. Treatment with high-dose thyroxine is effective in reducing recurrence.
D. Chemotherapy can be effective in the treatment of recurrence.
E. ^{131}I therapy can be used to treat local recurrence.
F. Block dissection of the lymph nodes in the neck is indicated.

1.23 Patients with morbid obesity:
- **A.** Need epidural PCA as the recommended method of analgesia.
- **B.** Are to be nursed sitting up postoperatively, to avoid hypoventilation and hypoxia.
- **C.** Require early mobilization.
- **D.** Have a higher rate of anaesthetic complications.
- **E.** Do not require thromboembolic deterrent stockings postoperatively.

1.24 Which of these statements is true about the healing of tubular bone fractures:
- **A.** The process of fracture healing starts with the fracture haematoma.
- **B.** Cell proliferation at the fracture site occurs late in the healing of fractures.
- **C.** The woven bone is transformed to lamellar bone by the osteoblasts.
- **D.** The callus at the fracture site is less profuse in children.
- **E.** Bone remodelling in children after a fracture is so perfect that eventually the site of the fracture becomes indistinguishable in radiographs.

1.25 The principal indications for percutaneous fine needle aspiration (FNA) cytopathology of the lung include:
- **A.** Suspected primary carcinoma in a patient considered to be suitable for thoracotomy.
- **B.** Suspected solitary or multiple lung metastases.
- **C.** Primary lung mass suspected as a source of metastases elsewhere.
- **D.** Suspected localized infectious process in which sputum or bronchoalveolar lavage has been negative.
- **E.** Suspected amyloidosis.

1.26 The following statements are true of acute osteomyelitis:
- **A.** It is common in children under the age of ten years.
- **B.** Positive blood cultures are rare.
- **C.** Streptococcal infection is the most common causative organism.
- **D.** A haematogenous source of the infection occurs in less than 25% of cases.
- **E.** High doses of systemic antibiotics are rarely effective.

1.27 Recognized complications of AIDS include:
 A. *Mycobacterium avium intracellulare* is a common secondary infection.
 B. Cytomegalovirus colitis.
 C. Enterocolitis caused by *Salmonella typhi*.
 D. Kaposi's sarcoma.
 E. Acute and chronic perianal sepsis.

1.28 Risk factors for deep vein thrombosis include:
 A. Antithrombin III deficiency.
 B. Nephrotic syndrome.
 C. Varicose veins.
 D. Hypotensive anaesthesia.
 E. Previous thrombophlebitis.
 F. Cancer.

1.29 The germination of tetanus spores in a wound is inhibited by:
 A. Tissue trauma.
 B. The presence of foreign bodies.
 C. Oxygen.
 D. An injection of antitoxin.
 E. An injection of toxoid.
 F. Surgical debridement of devitalized tissue.

1.30 *Clostridium tetani:*
 A. Causes gas gangrene.
 B. Produces an exotoxin.
 C. Has a terminal spore.
 D. Is an obligatory anaerobe.
 E. Is non-motile.

1.31 Prophylactic antibodies in surgery should be used for:
 A. Colorectal surgery.
 B. Breast reconstruction following mastectomy for cancer.
 C. Amputation.
 D. Patients with heart valve abnormalities.
 E. Total hip replacement.

1.32 The immunocompromised surgical patient may be:
A. HIV-positive.
B. A breast cancer patient with T2 N0 M0 disease.
C. A patient receiving four units of blood.
D. A patient with hypoxia.
E. Diabetic.

1.33 Factors adversely influencing wound healing and repair include:
A. Neoplasia.
B. Adhesions to bony surfaces.
C. Nephrotic syndrome.
D. Exposure to ionizing radiation.
E. Exposure to ultraviolet light.
F. Scurvy.

1.34 The body's response to trauma includes:
A. Vasoconstriction because of raised plasma levels of catecholamines.
B. Decreased glycogenolysis in the liver.
C. Increased secretions of insulin.
D. Increased plasma levels of glycerol.
E. Positive nitrogen balance.
F. Increased gluconeogenesis in the liver.

1.35 In postoperative pain relief:
A. Local anaesthetic infiltration significantly reduces the requirement for opioid analgesics.
B. Intramuscular opioid injection gives good and reliable uptake for pain relief.
C. Pethidine gives adequate analgesia for 4 h.
D. Oral analgesia should be given as soon as the pain is re-established.
E. Patient-controlled analgesia is effective in most elderly patients.

1.36 Diclofenac (Voltarol):
    A. Suppositories are useful analgesia in patients with Crohn's disease and ulcerative colitis.
    B. Is contraindicated in patients with asthma.
    C. Can be used in patients with epigastric pain and melaena.
    D. Is useful in a patient with ureteric colic in a dose of 75 mg b.d.
    E. Should be avoided in patients with renal impairment.

1.37 Acute visceral pain can be caused by:
    A. Cutting or burning of the hollow viscera.
    B. Distension of the hollow viscera.
    C. Ischaemia.
    D. Torsion or traction of the mesentery.
    E. Spasms of the smooth muscle of the hollow viscera.

1.38 Visceral pain:
    A. Can be exacerbated by eating and movement.
    B. Can be referred to distant regions of the body.
    C. Is represented by a large number of afferent fibres for small visceral areas.
    D. Is sharply localized to specific visceral regions.
    E. Is accompanied by powerful motor and autonomic reactions with increased sympathetic outflow.

1.39 The advantages of adding adrenaline to local anaesthetic are as follows:
    A. The total dose of local anaesthetic can be smaller.
    B. There is a slower systemic absorption of local anaesthetic.
    C. Longer action of local anaesthetic can be assured.
    D. There is less bleeding from the wound.
    E. It has no effect on healing in areas of poor tissue perfusion.

1.40 A 50-year-old woman develops severe right hypochondrial pain, pyrexia, rigors and hypotension 12 h after an ERCP and the removal of stones for choledocholithiasis:
  A. The patient is most likely suffering from pancreatitis.
  B. The most likely pathogenic cause of the sepsis is *Staphylococcus aureus*.
  C. The best antibiotic therapy is benzylpenicillin.
  D. She should be treated with an intravenous combination of gentamicin and metronidazole.
  E. Prophylactic antibiotics therapy would not prevent this complication of ERCP.
  F. An emergency repeat ERCP is advisable in the management of this patient.

1.41 A 60-year-old man is to undergo a low anterior resection for rectal cancer:
  A. He should receive subcutaneous heparin with premedication prior to an epidural analgesia to reduce the risks of post-operative complications.
  B. Antibiotic prophylaxis should be administered with his bowel preparation.
  C. Compartment pressure syndrome in the legs is a recognized complication.
  D. Intravenous fluids are given prior to surgery to avoid perioperative complications.
  E. Excess blood transfusion may cause further immunosuppression.

1.42 Pleural effusion in a postoperative patient following abdominal surgery can result from:
  A. Pneumonia.
  B. Congestive cardiac failure.
  C. Subdiaphragmatic abscess.
  D. Hypoalbuminaemia.
  E. Atelectasis.

1.43 Risk factors for developing abdominal incisional hernia include:
A. Diabetes.
B. Previous abdominal surgery.
C. Anaemia.
D. Hypoalbuminaemia.
E. Morbid obesity.
F. Intra-abdominal malignancy.

1.44 Postoperative pyrexia and sepsis:
A. Following a low anterior resection, this indicates an anastomotic leak until proven otherwise.
B. Can result from deep venous thrombosis and pulmonary embolism two days after surgery.
C. After two days may indicate a chest infection. ???
D. Following elective abdominal surgery are commonly an indication of subphrenic abscess.
E. Requires careful examination of the wound and rectal examination following elective abdominal surgery.

1.45 The following statements are true of wound infections:
A. *Staphylococcus aureus* is the most common organism to infect the surgical wound.
B. MRSA wound infection is usually the result of wound contamination by hospital staff.
C. Anaerobic organisms exert their lethal effects by producing endo- and exotoxins.
D. With opportunistic organisms, they are the result of a patient's reduced immune defence.
E. They frequently result in the development of incisional hernia.

1.46 Predisposing factors for the development of keloid scars include:
A. Patients of Afro-Caribbean origin with dark complexion.
B. Wound infection.
C. Steroid therapy.
D. Secondary wound closure.
E. Use of local bupivacaine.

1.47 The following statements regarding tracheostomy are correct:
- A. It is indicated in patients in need of long-term ventilation.
- B. It can only be performed as a cutdown procedure in the operating theatre.
- C. It requires formal surgical closure when it is no longer needed.
- D. The incision in the trachea is sited at the level of the second and third rings.
- E. It can help in weaning patients off a ventilator.
- F. Speech in such patients is prevented.
- G. It can lead to mechanical and infective complications unless scrupulous postoperative care is taken.

1.48 Deep venous thrombosis of the lower limb can be diagnosed by:
- A. A change in plasma viscosity.
- B. A Doppler ultrasound scan.
- C. Radioactive fibrinogen uptake.
- D. A positive Troisier's test.
- E. Venous thermogram.

1.49 Useful analgesics following a day surgery haemorrhoidectomy include:
- A. Slow-release morphine patches.
- B. Diclofenac.
- C. Local bupivacaine.
- D. Metronidazole therapy.
- E. Diamorphine.

1.50 These types of laser are recommended in the following surgical scenarios:
- A. An Argon laser is used for the avascular excision of tumours.
- B. A CO_2 laser is best for the photocoagulation of diabetic retinopathy.
- C. An Nd-YAG laser is used to arrest gastrointestinal bleeding.
- D. An Nd-YAG laser is of most use in palliative debulking of oesophageal tumours.
- E. A dye (tunable) photodynamic laser is used for the destruction of tumours after administration of a photosensitizing agent.

1.51 Theme: Lung masses

Options:
A. Abscess
B. Localized pneumonia
C. Tuberculosis
D. Pulmonary infarction
E. Primary carcinoma

For each of the patients described below, select the single most likely diagnosis from the list of options above. Each option may be used once, more than once or not at all.

1. A 45-year-old male – who is a heavy smoker – presented with cough, dyspnoea and haemoptysis of two weeks' duration.

2. A 28-year-old female presented with a cough and fever for three days, with dyspnoea on exertion. She smokes ten cigarettes a day.

3. A 71-year-old male comes into the outpatients' clinic with increasing shortness of breath, an irritating cough and weight loss (two stones) of two months' duration. History of tuberculosis treated 20 years previously.

1.52 Theme: Sterilization

Options:
A. Ethylene oxide
B. 160°C dry heat >120 minutes
C. Boiling
D. Gamma irradiation
E. Low temperature steam – 73°C for 20 min
F. High temperature steam – 134°C for 3 min

For each of the items described below, select the most suitable method of sterilization from the list of options above. Each option may be used once, more than once or not at all.

1. Laparoscopic surgical instruments.

2. Flexible endoscope.

3. Plastic syringes.

1.53 Theme: Assessment of risk for surgery

Options:
A. ASA 1
B. ASA 2
C. ASA 3
D. ASA
E. ASA 5
F. ASA 6

For each of the patients described below choose the most appropriate ASA status from those listed above. Each may be used once, more than once or not at all.

1. A 45-year-old smoker with known diabetes mellitus is booked for an elective inguinal hernia repair. He has a constant productive cough but is able to manage a flight of stairs. His diabetes is controlled with metformin.

2. A 60-year-old woman is admitted for an elective hysterectomy. At preoperative assessment she is found to have a blood pressure of 160/100 mmHg.

3. A 52-year-old man is admitted via the Accident and Emergency department complaining of severe central abdominal pain radiating to his back. He is hypotensive and sweaty. A CXR shows no air under the diaphragm. After resuscitation with intravenous fluids a pulsatile mass is felt in his abdomen.

CORE MODULE **2**

Perioperative management (II)

2.1 Insulin dependent diabetic patients:
A. Are at risk of cerebrovascular disease.
B. Require preoperative lying and standing blood pressure measurement.
C. Need hourly perioperative monitoring of urinary glucose.
D. Are less prone to sepsis postoperatively.
E. Should be resuscitated with Hartmann's solution.

2.2 Indications for a routine preoperative chest X-ray include:
A. A patient of more than 50 years of age.
B. Surgery for benign disease.
C. Emphysema.
D. Asthma.
E. Laparoscopic surgery.

2.3 Before referring a patient for magnetic resonance imaging (MRI) the physician should determine:
A. If the patient is agoraphobic.
B. If a pacemaker has been inserted.
C. If surgical clips are in place.
D. If the patient has sustained an eye injury.
E. If the patient is allergic to iodine containing compounds.

2.4 Preoperative sickle cell testing should be considered:
A. In Anglo-Saxon patients.
B. In Afro-Caribbeans.
C. In South Americans.
D. In Hispanics.
E. In Indians.

2.5 Preoperative ECG recordings are needed in:
A. Hypertensive patients.
B. Patients over the age of 50.
C. Diabetic patients.
D. Patients who smoke.
E. Patients suspected of having Addison's disease.

2.6 Fresh frozen plasma:
A. Contains Factor VIII.
B. Is used in the treatment of disseminated intravascular coagulopathy.
C. Is used for the reversal of warfarin.
D. Is prepared from pooled donation.
E. May transmit Hepatitis C.

2.7 In colorectal surgery, antibiotic prophylaxis:
A. Significantly reduces the risk of postoperative wound infection.
B. With metronidazole alone is sufficient to reduce superficial wound infection.
C. With new second-generation cephalosporins is more efficacious than first generation.
D. Should continue for at least three days.
E. Should be universally agreed throughout UK hospitals.

2.8 Superficial abscesses:
A. Are commonly caused by *Staphylococcus aureus*.
B. In the perianal region should be treated conservatively.
C. Of the breast are best drained through horizontal incisions.
D. Require drainage and treatment with antibiotics.
E. Begin as an accumulation of macrophages around a bacterial innoculum.

2.9 Universal precautions used in the treatment of high risk patients include:
A. The use of blunt needles.
B. Exhaust body suits.
C. Waterproof footwear.
D. Hand to hand passing of sharps.
E. Double glove techniques.

2.10 Monopolar surgical diathermy:
A. Is an alternating current in the range 40–60 kHz.
B. Results in temperatures of up to 1000°C.
C. Requires a patient electrode of at least 70 cm².
D. Should not be used in the presence of a pacemaker.
E. Cannot be used for 'cutting'.

2.11 The Nd-YAG laser:
A. Is a beam of coherent dichromatic electromagnetic radiation.
B. Is derived from a gaseous medium.
C. Is in the invisible infra-red light range.
D. Causes minimal scarring.
E. Routes light via a series of mirrors.

2.12 Thrombocytopaenia may result from:
A. Hyposplenism.
B. Disseminated intravascular coagulation.
C. Lymphoma.
D. Steroid treatment.
E. Bone marrow infiltration.

2.13 Hypertensive patients undergoing surgery are at risk of:
A. Renal disease.
B. Deep venous thrombosis.
C. Myocardial infarction.
D. Disseminated intravascular coagulation.
E. Cerebrovascular accident.

2.14 Morbidly obese patients undergoing abdominal surgery:
A. Are more prone to wound infection.
B. Are prone to hypocapnia.
C. Are three times the ideal weight for their height.
D. May develop exacerbation of arthritis.
E. Should not be operated on laparoscopically.

2.15 Postoperative complications in patients with obstructive jaundice may be prevented by:
A. The use of intravenous steroids perioperatively.
B. Adequate intravenous hydration.
C. Biliary stenting.
D. The administration of 200 ml of 50% mannitol perioperatively.
E. Correction of prothrombin time with oral Vitamin K.

2.16 Rates of postoperative wound infection may be minimized by:
   A. 'Scrubbing' for 5 min between each case.
   B. Reducing the number of personnel in the operating theatre.
   C. Meticulous haemostasis.
   D. The use of braided sutures.
   E. Wearing theatre masks.

2.17 In minor surgical procedures:
   A. Incisions should be made perpendicular to the skin tension lines.
   B. An advancement flap is the best technique for lengthening a contracted scar.
   C. The spinal accessory nerve is at risk in the anterior triangle of the neck.
   D. Infected wounds may be left open.
   E. Keloid scarring extends beyond the original excision scar.

2.18 Keloid scars:
   A. Are distinguished from hypertrophic scars by their extent.
   B. Occur more frequently in pigmented skin.
   C. Are caused by the excess deposition of fibrin in the wound.
   D. Are common on the deltoid region.
   E. May be prevented by pressure dressings.

2.19 A clean contaminated operation:
   A. Is defined as one including the controlled opening of any hollow viscus.
   B. Is associated with a 15% risk of postoperative infection.
   C. Requires five days' prophylaxis with antibiotics.
   D. May predispose to systemic inflammatory response syndrome.
   E. May include stoma formation.

2.20 The following factors increase the likelihood of postoperative sepsis:
- A. Immunosuppression.
- B. Obesity.
- C. Emergency.
- D. Length of preoperative stay.
- E. Rough handling of tissue during surgery.

2.21 *Staphylococcus aureus* is sensitive to:
- A. Vancomycin.
- B. Cefuroxime.
- C. Flucloxacillin.
- D. Clindamycin.
- E. Methicillin.

2.22 Endogenous infections:
- A. Are reduced by the use of broad-spectrum antibiotics preoperatively.
- B. May be prevented by the use of laminar air flow in theatres.
- C. May be transmitted by affected healthcare workers.
- D. Arise from organisms acquired in hospital.
- E. Are commonly caused by Gram-negative organisms.

2.23 In the perioperative period patients may become immunocompromised as a result of:
- A. Jaundice.
- B. Congenital hypergammaglobulinaemia.
- C. Salazopyrine.
- D. Splenectomy.
- E. HIV infection.

2.24 During a right hemicolectomy:
- A. A round-bodied needle is used for suturing the skin.
- B. A reverse cutting needle is used for any bowel anastomosis.
- C. A blunt needle may be used for mass closure of the wound.
- D. Wound dehiscence is more likely if an absorbable suture is used for mass closure.
- E. A J needle is employed for a subcuticular suture.

2.25 Leakage of a bowel anastomosis should be suspected if:
- **A.** The patient develops a pyrexia.
- **B.** Free gas is found under the diaphragm ten days' postoperatively.
- **C.** The patient has frequent watery stool.
- **D.** Bloodstained pus discharges through the vagina.
- **E.** Abdominal distension develops.

2.26 T-tube drains:
- **A.** Are only used in the biliary tree.
- **B.** Are made of silastic rubber.
- **C.** Should be removed after seven days.
- **D.** May cause peritonitis when they are removed from the common bile duct.
- **E.** Are easily occluded.

2.27 A posterolateral thoracotomy in the 5th intercostal space:
- **A.** Is at the level of the lung hilum.
- **B.** Provides access to the great vessels.
- **C.** Is limited posteriorly by the intervertebral muscles.
- **D.** Should be made along the inferior border of the rib.
- **E.** Is closed using No. 1 vicryl sutures.

2.28 Lignocaine:
- **A.** Inhibits the uptake of sodium into nerve cell membranes.
- **B.** Has a local vasodilatory effect.
- **C.** Toxicity should be suspected if the patient develops slurred speech.
- **D.** Is an alkaline solution.
- **E.** 1% solution contains 1 g of lignocaine in 100 ml fluid.

2.29 Local anaesthetic injections are less painful if:
- **A.** The anaesthetic is cooled.
- **B.** They are combined with adrenaline.
- **C.** They are given rapidly.
- **D.** The acid pH is neutralized prior to administration.
- **E.** A thinner needle is used.

2.30 Theme: Investigations

Options:
A. Erect CXR
B. BM Stix
C. Amylase
D. Abdominal CT
E. Abdominal ultrasound
F. Arterial blood gases
G. ECG

From the list above choose the single test most likely to confirm your clinical suspicion for the patients listed below. Each answer may be used once, more than once or not at all.

1. A 54-year-old woman presents to the Accident and Emergency department with a one-week history of upper abdominal pain. The pain is colicky in nature and exacerbated by meals. Initial blood tests show Hb 12; WBC 10.9; platelets 243; bilirubin 35; alkaline phosphatase 280; AST 50.

2. A 25-year-old female patient complains of sudden onset of chest pain one week after nailing of a femoral fracture sustained in a road traffic accident. On examination she is pyrexial and has an elevated respiratory rate.

2.31 Theme: Infecting organisms

Options:
A. Aerobic Gram-positive cocci
B. Aerobic Gram-positive rod
C. Aerobic Gram-negative cocci
D. Aerobic Gram-negative rod
E. Facultative Gram-positive cocci
F. Facultative Gram-positive rod
G. Facultative Gram-negative cocci
H. Facultative Gram-negative rod

From the list above choose the correct classification of the organisms listed below. Each answer may be used once, more than once or not at all.

1. *Clostridium botulinum.*

2. Campylobacter species.

3. *Escherichia coli.*

2.32 Theme: Infection

Options:
A. *Streptococcus viridans*
B. *Escherichia coli*
C. *Streptococcus pneumoniae*
D. *Mycobacterium* tuberculosis
E. *Streptococcus milleri*
F. *Bacillus cereus*
G. *Clostridium difficile*
H. *Clostridium perfringens*
I. *Clostridium tetani*
J. *Streptococcus pyogenes*

For each of the infections listed below choose the most likely pathogen from the list above. Each answer may be used once, more than once or not at all.

1. Community acquired respiratory tract infection.

2. Necrotizing fasciitis.

3. Cerebral abscess.

2.33 Theme: Biopsy techniques

Options:
A. Incisional biopsy
B. Fine needle aspiration
C. Core needle biopsy
D. Brush cytology
E. Endoscopic biopsy
F. Excisional biopsy

From the list above choose the most appropriate first-line biopsy technique for the lesions listed below. Each answer may be used once, more than once or not at all.

1. Solitary breast lump.

2. Suspected skin melanoma.

3. Biliary stricture.

Trauma

3.1 During initial assessment of the multiply injured patient, the following are true:
A. Shock management is the first priority.
B. Cervical spine control is usually necessary.
C. External haemorrhage should be ignored.
D. Pulse oximetry is usually unhelpful.
E. Ischaemic limbs demand immediate attention.

3.2 Regarding management of the airway in the multiply injured patient:
A. High concentrations of oxygen should initially be avoided.
B. Airway obstruction is usually caused by a foreign body.
C. The oropharyngeal airway is well tolerated in semiconscious patients.
D. The laryngeal mask airway protects against tracheobronchial aspiration.
E. The endotracheal tube can only be passed in spontaneously breathing patients.

3.3 The following features are seen in the adult patient who has acutely lost 750 ml of blood:
A. Mild tachycardia.
B. Reduced blood pressure.
C. Oliguria.
D. Pallor with diminished capillary refill.
E. An acute fall in haematocrit.

3.4 The patient with tension pneumothorax will exhibit the following:
A. Tachypnoea.
B. Agitation.
C. Decreased percussion note on the injured side.
D. Collapsed neck veins.
E. Decreased chest wall movement on the injured side.

3.5 The following chest injuries are immediately life threatening:

A. Tension pneumothorax.
B. Open pneumothorax.
C. Ruptured diaphragm.
D. Pulmonary contusion.
E. Flail chest.

3.6 The following chest injuries respond well to ventilation:

A. Tension pneumothorax.
B. Flail chest.
C. Open pneumothorax.
D. Ruptured diaphragm.
E. Pulmonary contusion.

3.7 Chest drain insertion is usually indicated in patients with the following:

A. Mediastinal traversing wounds.
B. Flail chest.
C. Open pneumothorax.
D. Ruptured diaphragm.
E. Surgical emphysema.

3.8 Resuscitative thoracotomy is indicated in patients with the following:

A. Penetrating chest injuries (who are pulseless).
B. Penetrating chest injuries (who are stable).
C. Blunt chest injuries (pulseless).
D. Massive haemothorax, that is, more than 1500 ml blood in the chest cavity.
E. Cardiac tamponade (stable).

3.9 Regarding diagnostic peritoneal lavage, the following statements are true:

A. The bladder should first be catheterized.
B. Initial aspirate of blood is deemed to be positive.
C. 20 ml/kg of saline is used for lavage.
D. Greater than 1000 red cells per mm^3 is deemed to be positive.
E. Greater than 500 white cells per mm^3 is deemed to be positive.

3.10 In the alert patient with evidence of blunt abdominal trauma:
- A. Peritoneal lavage is helpful if the patient is stable.
- B. Peritoneal lavage is indicated if the patient is unstable.
- C. CT scanning can usually exclude serious intra-abdominal injury.
- D. CT scanning will visualize retroperitoneal injuries well.
- E. Laparotomy is usually necessary in the shocked patient.

3.11 In the patient with a single gunshot wound to the abdomen:
- A. Peritoneal lavage is helpful in the management of the stable patient.
- B. CT scanning can usually exclude serious intra-abdominal injury.
- C. Splenic injuries are more common than bowel injuries.
- D. Laparotomy is invariably indicated.
- E. Strict cervical spine control must be maintained.

3.12 Regarding pelvic fractures, the following statements are true:
- A. Pelvic fractures are usually detectable by clinical examination alone.
- B. Diagnostic peritoneal lavage is more likely to be falsely positive.
- C. Skeletal fixation often reduces pelvic haemorrhage.
- D. An associated rectal laceration renders the pelvic fracture open.
- E. Peritoneal lavage should be performed above the umbilicus.

3.13 The following statements are true:
- A. Normal intracranial pressure (ICP) is approximately 10 mmHg.
- B. ICP can remain normal despite a space-occupying lesion.
- C. Cerebral perfusion pressure is independent of ICP.
- D. Hypotensive patients tend to have a low ICP.
- E. Autoregulation refers to maintenance of constant cerebral blood flow.

3.14 The following statements are true:
A. The precentral gyrus controls motor function.
B. Compression of the oculomotor nerve causes pupillary constriction.
C. The corticospinal tract crosses to the opposite side at tentorial level.
D. CSF is absorbed into the superior sagittal sinus via the choroid plexus.
E. The posterior cranial fossa houses the occipital lobes.

3.15 Regarding acute extradural haematoma, the following are true:
A. Patients usually have ipsilateral pupillary dilatation.
B. Patients usually have contralateral hemiplegia.
C. CT demonstrates a biconvex lesion.
D. Bleeding can be from arterial or venous sources.
E. A lucid interval is sometimes seen.

3.16 The following statements are true:
A. The prognosis for extradural haematoma is worse than subdural haematoma.
B. Subdural haematomas usually occur from a venous source.
C. A skull vault fracture significantly increases the risk of intracranial haematoma.
D. A basal skull fracture significantly increases the risk of intracranial haematoma.
E. An open skull fracture implies the dura mater is torn.

3.17 When managing a patient with head injury:
A. Intubation is usually required in patients with a GCS less than 13.
B. Hyperventilation is required to improve oxygenation.
C. Hypotension indicates a loss of autoregulation.
D. Skull X-rays are valuable for initial management.
E. Pupillary signs are unreliable following anaesthesia for intubation.

3.18 **The following statements are true:**
   A. The spinal cord terminates at the L4 level.
   B. The spinothalamic tract transmits pain and temperature sensation from the opposite side of the body.
   C. The posterior column transmits position sense and touch sensation from the same side of the body.
   D. The C7 dermatome innervates thumb sensation.
   E. The L3 myotome innervates knee extension.

3.19 **In the initial presentation of low cervical spinal cord injury:**
   A. Hypotension and bradycardia usually indicate blood loss.
   B. There is unlikely to be respiratory abnormality.
   C. Sacral sparing of sensation is associated with a better prognosis.
   D. Lower limb spasticity and hyperreflexia is usually seen.
   E. High dose steroids have no effect on outcome.

3.20 **Concerning trauma scoring systems:**
   A. The abbreviated injury scale can be used as a field triage tool.
   B. The injury severity score is a measure of physiological disturbance.
   C. The revised trauma score utilizes GCS, systolic blood pressure and respiratory rate.
   D. TRISS methodology provides a statistical measure of probability of survival.
   E. APACHE II scoring takes chronic ill-health into account.

3.21 **The following statements regarding skin grafting are true:**
   A. A split-skin graft involves approximately 50% of epidermal thickness.
   B. A skin graft normally 'takes' within 24 h of grafting.
   C. Muscle normally provides a suitable bed for split-skin grafting.
   D. The presence of *Staphylococcus aureus* will usually result in graft failure.
   E. A split-skin graft can be stored for several weeks before application.

3.22 The following statements regarding flaps are true:
A. A flap describes composite tissue transfer with maintenance of vascular network.
B. A full thickness skin graft is the simplest form of flap.
C. A pedicled flap re-establishes local blood supply in about three weeks.
D. A free flap describes one that does not result in a secondary defect.
E. A TRAM flap describes a composite fibular transfer used to replace areas of bone loss.

3.23 The following statements regarding burns are true:
A. Full thickness burns are not normally associated with blistering.
B. Superficial partial thickness burns normally heal within ten days.
C. Wallace's Rule of Nines refers to a fluid replacement formula.
D. Thermal injury to the airways often results in bronchospasm.
E. Carboxyhaemoglobinaemia will not be detected by a pulse oximeter.
F. Burns normally require antibiotic prophylaxis against Streptococcal infection.

3.24 Regarding maxillary fractures, the following statements are correct:
A. A Le Fort 1 fracture involves damage to the orbital skeleton.
B. CSF rhinorrhoea is commonly seen in association with high maxillary fractures.
C. Such patients require intubation by the nasal route rather than oral route.
D. An orthopantomogram visualizes maxillary fractures well.
E. Occipitomental X-rays are best obtained with a supine patient.

3.25 Orbital blowout fractures:
  A. Can occur through the medial orbit or inferior orbit.
  B. Are often associated with damage to the ophthalmic nerve.
  C. Cause diplopia by interference with oculomotor nerve function.
  D. Are often associated with infraorbital paraesthesia.
  E. Are clearly demonstrated by axial CT scans.

3.26 The following statements concerning gunshot wounds are true:
  A. Temporary cavitation is caused by a sonic shock wave in high velocity injuries.
  B. Solid organs such as liver resist cavitation more than softer tissue such as lung.
  C. High velocity injuries usually have less bacterial contamination.
  D. Abdominal gunshot wounds invariably require laparotomy.
  E. Cranial gunshot wounds invariably require ventilation.

3.27 During a major incident the following terms are commonly employed:
  A. The Primary Triage Officer is an ambulance officer at the scene.
  B. At the hospital the Chief Triage Officer is normally an experienced A and E nurse.
  C. The 'expectant' triage category denotes those with minor injuries.
  D. Patients who are not breathing despite airway manoeuvres are prioritized for immediate care.
  E. The Medical Incident Officer controls the hospital response.

3.28 Regarding wound management, the following statements are true:

A. Primary closure should not normally be carried out on wounds more than 6 h old.

B. Healing by second intention is useful for dirty facial wounds.

C. Radiographs of wounds which contain glass will be positive in around 50% of cases.

D. Antibiotics are normally required for hand lacerations.

E. The commonest organism to infect skin wounds is *Streptococcus pyogenes*.

3.29 The following statements are true:

A. The median nerve supplies the interossei of the hand.

B. The radial nerve supplies abductor pollicis brevis.

C. The ulnar nerve supplies sensation to the one-and-a-half ulnar digits.

D. The radial nerve supplies all extensor muscles of the forearm.

E. The biceps muscle is supplied by the musculocutaneous nerve.

3.30 The following statements are true:

A. The femoral nerve supplies all of the quadriceps muscle.

B. A superficial peroneal nerve injury will result in foot drop.

C. A common peroneal nerve injury will produce loss of sensation to all interdigital clefts.

D. The tibial nerve supplies all the ankle and digital flexors.

E. The sciatic nerve is prone to injury during posterior hip dislocation.

3.31 The following statements regarding fracture healing are true:
A. A spiral fracture will heal faster than a transverse fracture.
B. A comminuted fracture will heal faster than a transverse fracture.
C. A diaphyseal (midshaft) injury will heal faster than a metaphyseal injury.
D. Rigid internal fixation usually results in more rapid fracture healing.
E. In children epiphyseal injuries usually heal faster than non-epiphyseal injuries.

3.32 The following situations often lead to delayed fracture union:
A. Fractures where there is joint involvement.
B. Fractures of osteoporotic bone.
C. Fractures in the elderly.
D. Compound fractures.
E. Excessive mobility at the fracture site.

3.33 The following statements are true:
A. Hip stiffness is commonly seen after femoral fractures.
B. Avascular necrosis is often seen in the distal scaphoid.
C. Avascular necrosis is sometimes seen in the head of the talus.
D. Fat embolism classically occurs 7–10 days after injury.
E. Compartment syndrome is always accompanied by loss of distal pulses.

3.34 Theme: Airway management

Options:
A. Supplemental oxygen alone
B. Supplemental oxygen with an oropharyngeal airway
C. Supplemental oxygen with a nasopharyngeal airway
D. Supplemental oxygen with laryngeal mask airway
E. Orotracheal intubation and IPPV
F. Nasotracheal intubation and IPPV
G. Cricothyroidotomy and IPPV

For each of the patients described below, select the single most appropriate management from the list of options above. Each option may be used once, more than once or not at all.

1. A 25-year-old man (X) is brought to the emergency department following a closed head injury. There is no evidence of extracranial injury, and the patient is breathing spontaneously. He is however deeply comatose with a GCS of 5 and there is evidence of CSF rhinorrhoea and periorbital bruising. How should his airway be managed?

2. A 45-year-old man (Y) is brought to the emergency department following blunt trauma to the head and face. There is no evidence of extracranial injury, but the airway is clearly obstructed. The patient is deeply comatose with a GCS of 4 and there are obvious grossly displaced facial fractures. Visualization of the pharynx is obscured because of fracture displacement and bleeding. How should the airway be managed?

3.35 Theme: Abdominal trauma management

Options:
A. Observation
B. Ultrasound
C. CT scan
D. Diagnostic peritoneal lavage (DPL)
E. Immediate laparotomy

For each of the patients described below, select the single most appropriate management from the list of options above. Each option may be used once, more than once or not at all.

1. A 50-year-old car driver (X), is injured following a high speed road traffic accident. He is conscious on admission to the emergency department but is clearly haemodynamically unstable. He has marked abdominal tenderness. The trauma series of X-rays (cervical spine, chest and pelvis) are normal, and secondary survey reveals no other abnormality. How should you proceed to manage his abdominal injury?

2. A 23-year-old man (Y) is stabbed in the right upper quadrant of the abdomen. This appears to be an isolated injury and he is stable on admission to the emergency department. Abdominal examination reveals only mild local tenderness. How will you manage this patient's abdominal injury?

3. A 32-year-old woman (Z) is admitted to the emergency department with multiple injuries. She has multiple rib fractures with a moderate haemothorax, is deeply comatose, and has bilateral femoral fractures. Initial management includes endotracheal intubation, chest drainage and fluid infusion. The c-spine and pelvis X-rays are normal. She is haemodynamically very unstable. How should you manage the possibility of abdominal injury?

3.36 Theme: Chest injuries

Options:
A. Perform needle thoracentesis
B. Insert a chest drain
C. Perform a chest X-ray
D. Obtain arterial blood gases
E. Obtain a CT of chest
F. Proceed to emergency room thoracotomy

For each of the patients described below, select the single most appropriate management from the list of options above. Each option may be used once, more than once or not at all.

1. A 33-year-old man sustains a gunshot wound to the right hemithorax, with entry in the 4th intercostal space and exit through the axilla. He is mildly shocked but is receiving fluid infusion. He is otherwise stable and is conscious and co-operative. Chest examination reveals slightly diminished air entry with dullness at the posterior chest. What is your next step in management of this chest injury?

2. An elderly man falls at home sustaining multiple rib fractures. He is in obvious discomfort but generally stable. His chest X-ray reveals single fractures of five ribs on the right side, and a very small (10%) pneumothorax. What should you do next to manage his chest injury?

Intensive care

4.1 **In the AP chest X-ray:**
  A. The right diaphragm normally lies at the level of the lower border of the 7th rib anteriorly.
  B. The carina lies at the level of the 2nd thoracic vertebra behind the sternal angle.
  C. The left hilum is normally slightly higher than the right.
  D. The horizontal fissure can be traced from the mid-axillary line at the level of the 4th rib horizontally across the chest wall.
  E. The aortic valve lies above the mitral valve.

4.2 **The following statements concerning lung volumes are true:**
  A. The lung is composed of four volumes and four capacities.
  B. FRC = inspiratory reserve volume + tidal volume.
  C. Vital capacity = total lung capacity – residual volume.
  D. FRC falls with age.
  E. FRC increases with obesity.

4.3 **The 12-lead ECG:**
  A. Has a normal running speed of 50 mm/s.
  B. Has a normal gain of 1 cm to 1 mV.
  C. Has a normal PR interval of 0.12–0.20 s.
  D. Could indicate a complete bundle branch block with a QRS complex duration of more than 0.12 s.
  E. Has a normal axis of – 90° to + 90°.

4.4   The pulmonary artery floatation catheter:
A. May precipitate complete heart block in patients with LBBB.
B. Is useful for sampling mixed venous blood.
C. Has a proximal lumen that opens into the right ventricle.
D. Gives accurate wedge pressures in the presence of pulmonary hypertension.
E. Is useful in differentiating between right and left-sided cardiac failure.

4.5.   Complications following a 700 ml blood transfusion in a fit 70 kg adult male are likely to include:
A. Hyperkalaemia.
B. Air embolism.
C. Haemolytic anaemia.
D. Metabolic acidosis.
E. Thrombophlebitis.

4.6   An increase in the $P_AO_2{:}P_aO_2$ gradient is seen:
A. In the supine position.
B. Following opioid medication.
C. On addition of PEEP.
D. Following upper abdominal incisions.
E. When shivering.

4.7   Spirometry may be used to measure:
A. Functional residual capacity.
B. Tidal volume.
C. Inspiratory reserve volume.
D. Total lung capacity.
E. Vital capacity.

4.8   Pulse oximetry may give inaccurate readings in:
A. Jaundice.
B. Shock.
C. Smokers.
D. The presence of nail varnish.
E. Excessively darkened rooms.

4.9 Functional residual capacity (FRC) may be estimated using:
  A. Nitrogen washout.
  B. Fowler's method.
  C. Helium dilution.
  D. Body plethysmography.
  E. The Bohr equation.

4.10 A paralysed patient may be ventilated using:
  A. Intermittent positive pressure ventilation (IPPV).
  B. Positive end-expiratory pressure (PEEP).
  C. Pressure support ventilation (PSV).
  D. Synchronized intermittent mandatory ventilation (SIMV).
  E. Continuous positive airways pressure (CPAP).

4.11 Intravenous dopamine:
  A. Does not cross the blood–brain barrier.
  B. Increases the cardiac output.
  C. Is antiemetic.
  D. Causes vasoconstriction of the splanchnic vascular bed.
  E. Increases urine output.

4.12 Dextrose/saline (dextrose 4% and saline 0.18%) 1 l:
  A. Contains 62 mmol sodium ions.
  B. Contains 41 mmol chloride ions.
  C. Has a calculated osmolality of 250 mosmol/l.
  D. Has an energy content of approximately 150 kcal.
  E. Has a pH of 4.5.

4.13 Typical fluid and electrolyte and nutritional replacement over a 24 h period in a 70 kg starved patient (with no other overt losses) could include:
  A. 2700 ml water.
  B. 70 mmol sodium.
  C. 70 mmol potassium.
  D. 3000 kcal energy.
  E. 70 g protein.

4.14 Causes of hyponatraemia include:
A. Hyperlipidaemia.
B. Hepatic cirrhosis.
C. Lithium therapy.
D. Diarrhoea.
E. Diabetes insipidus.

4.15 Concerning sedation in the intensive care unit:
A. Midazolam has a short elimination half-life.
B. Morphine is metabolized by the liver.
C. Pethidine has no active metabolites.
D. The Ramsay score is a useful index of sedative level.
E. Fentanyl is a water-soluble analgesic.

4.16 Salicylate poisoning may present with:
A. Respiratory acidosis.
B. Metabolic acidosis.
C. Hypokalaemia.
D. Fever.
E. Tinnitus.

4.17 Concerning carbon monoxide (CO) poisoning:
A. Carbon monoxide has a lower affinity for haemoglobin binding than oxygen.
B. Carboxyhaemoglobin (COHb) level correlates well with symptoms and severity.
C. Hyperbaric oxygen therapy is indicated for patients with neurological impairment.
D. Arterial oxygen concentration (P_aO_2) is reduced.
E. CO poisoning may result in delayed neuropsychiatric problems.

4.18 In patients presenting with acute spinal cord injuries:
A. High-dose methylprednisolone therapy is indicated within 8 h.
B. Vasoconstriction, hypertension and tachycardia are seen.
C. Twenty per cent of patients have an associated head injury.
D. Hyperbaric oxygen therapy improves long-term outcome.
E. There is an increased risk of deep venous thrombo-embolism.

4.19 Tetanus:
A. Is caused by the endotoxin tetanospasmin produced by *Clostridium tetani*.
B. Has an incubation period ranging from 2–60 days.
C. May be treated using human tetanus immunoglobulin.
D. May produce severe cardiovascular disturbances.
E. Produces immunity for those who survive an initial infection.

4.20 The following statements are true of drugs affecting renal function:
A. Dopamine increases sodium reabsorption in the tubular cell.
B. Dobutamine causes renal vasodilatation.
C. Caffeine is a weak diuretic.
D. Aminoglycosides are toxic to the proximal tubule.
E. Loop diuretics act in the descending loop of Henle.

4.21 Vancomycin:
A. Is a broad-spectrum antibiotic.
B. Is active against methicillin-resistant *Staph. Aureus* (MRSA).
C. Commonly produces nephrotoxicity.
D. May cause Red Man syndrome.
E. Is indicated in treatment of antibiotic associated colitis.

4.22 In cases of near drowning:
A. The extent of lung injury depends largely on the volume of water aspirated.
B. Steroids are indicated in treatment of brain oedema associated with near drowning.
C. Prophylactic antibiotic coverage is not indicated.
D. Hypoglycaemia is common.
E. Hypernatraemia and hyperchloraemia may occur in saltwater near drowning cases.

4.23 ECG changes associated with hyperkalaemia include:
A. High peaked T waves.
B. Narrow QRS interval.
C. Prolonged QT interval.
D. Sine wave.
E. ST segment depression.

4.24 Cerebral blood flow:
A. Is approximately 50 ml/100 g/min.
B. Is subject to autoregulation.
C. Decreases with hyperkalaemia.
D. Is increased by 4% for each 0.1 kPa rise in P_aCO_2.
E. May be determined clinically by transcranial Doppler measurement.

4.25 The intra-aortic balloon pump:
A. Increases cardiac output by increasing systemic vascular resistance.
B. Increases coronary artery perfusion pressure.
C. May be used in the treatment of cardiogenic shock.
D. May be triggered by P waves on the ECG.
E. Is contraindicated in patients with severe aortic regurgitation.

4.26 Metabolic acidosis may result in:
A. Potassium retention.
B. Elevation of plasma chloride.
C. Lowering of P_aCO_2.
D. Tetany.
E. Reduction in plasma phosphate.

4.27 For a diagnosis of brain death the following criteria must be met:
A. Flat EEG.
B. Absent motor responses.
C. Absent respiratory efforts despite P_aCO_2 of 6.6 kPa.
D. Presence of 'doll's eyes' movement for the oculocephalic reflex.
E. The doctor making the diagnosis must have been registered for five years.

4.28 Rhabdomyolysis:
A. May occur without a history of trauma.
B. Is frequently associated with hypercalcaemia in the acute phase.
C. Is frequently associated with hyperkalaemia in the acute phase.
D. Is treated with large volume fluid resuscitation.
E. Is associated with a rise in plasma CPK.

4.29 In Adult Respiratory Distress Syndrome (ARDS):
   A. Lung oedema occurs because of increased hydrostatic pressure.
   B. Pancreatitis may coexist.
   C. Nitric oxide is of proven benefit.
   D. Pulmonary compliance is reduced.
   E. Surfactant function is disturbed.

4.30 An elderly woman is dehydrated from a prolonged intestinal obstruction. She is tachypnoeic and distressed, breathing air. The following are likely:
   A. Respiratory alkalosis.
   B. Metabolic acidosis.
   C. Hypoxaemia.
   D. Uraemia.
   E. Hyperglycaemia.

4.31 Hypotension and an elevated central venous pressure may occur in:
   A. Pulmonary embolism.
   B. Haemorrhage.
   C. Congestive cardiac failure.
   D. Myocardial infarction.
   E. Tension pneumothorax.

4.32 The following may be features of the transurethral resection (TUR) syndrome:
   A. Hypotension and tachycardia.
   B. Confusion.
   C. Hyponatraemia.
   D. Haemolysis.
   E. Disseminated intravascular coagulation.

4.33 Fat embolism can cause:
   A. Central cyanosis.
   B. A petechial rash.
   C. Hypoventilation.
   D. Cerebral oedema.
   E. Pyrexia.

4.34 The following may cause a metabolic alkalosis:
A. Cushing syndrome.
B. Gastrocolic fistula.
C. Hyperkalaemia.
D. Pyloric stenosis.
E. Acetazolamide therapy.

4.35 An arterial line in the radial artery can lead to:
A. Pulmonary embolism.
B. Fatal haemorrhage.
C. Intracerebral embolism.
D. Paraesthesia at the base of the thumb.
E. Septicaemia.

4.36 In an unconscious patient the following clinical signs suggest a cervical cord injury:
A. Hypotension with bradycardia.
B. Diaphragmatic breathing.
C. Priapism.
D. Flaccid arreflexia of the limbs.
E. A fixed, dilated pupil.

4.37 Disseminated intravascular coagulation (DIC) may occur in:
A. Amniotic fluid embolus.
B. Acute promyelocytic leukaemia.
C. *Falciparum* malaria.
D. Haemolytic transfusion reaction.
E. Thrombotic thrombocytopenic purpura.

4.38 In acute liver failure:
A. A prothrombin time > 20 s indicates severe failure.
B. The level of serum alanine aminotransferase (LDH) is a sensitive marker.
C. The serum bilirubin is a sensitive marker.
D. Paracetamol may be implicated aetiologically.
E. Halothane may be implicated aetiologically.

4.39 The oxyhaemoglobin dissociation curve:
A. Is shifted to the right in chronic anaemia.
B. Is shifted to the left in the pulmonary capillaries.
C. Is shifted to the left in hypoventilation.
D. Is unaffected by temperature.
E. Is shifted to the right in carbon monoxide poisoning.

4.40 Vomiting may be associated with:
  A. Metabolic alkalosis.
  B. Alkaline urine.
  C. Raised plasma chloride levels.
  D. Hyperkalaemia.
  E. Elevated blood urea.

4.41 In electrocardiography:
  A. A potassium ion gradient is mainly responsible for the electrical potential difference across the cell membrane.
  B. An exploring electrode records an upward deflection when the depolarization current is flowing away from it.
  C. The PR interval is reduced in first degree heart block.
  D. The QT interval is reduced in hypocalcaemia.
  E. The T wave is caused by ventricular repolarization.

4.42 Immediate problems post thyroidectomy include:
  A. Tracheal stenosis.
  B. Wound haematoma.
  C. Hypocalcaemia.
  D. Thyroid crisis.
  E. Laryngeal stridor.

4.43 With effective cardiopulmonary resuscitation:
  A. An inspired oxygen concentration of about 14% can be produced using mouth to mouth.
  B. The patient's expired CO_2 will be less than 2%.
  C. Acidosis will be prevented.
  D. Arterial pH will approach 7.4.
  E. A mixed venous haemoglobin saturation of 85% is likely.

4.44 Mannitol:
  A. Is an alcohol.
  B. May be used to prevent the hepatorenal syndrome in jaundiced patients.
  C. Should not be coadministered with blood.
  D. Is hypertonic.
  E. May cause a rise in intracranial pressure.

4.45 Bronchospasm:
A. May be caused by morphine.
B. May be caused by pethidine.
C. May be caused by irritation from the endotracheal tube.
D. Can produce similar physical signs to cardiac failure.
E. Is exacerbated by the volatile agent halothane.

4.46 Basal metabolic rate (BMR):
A. Is increased with propofol.
B. Is increased by 1.4% for every °C rise in temperature.
C. Remains unaffected by exercise.
D. Is affected by age.
E. Is increased with pain.

4.47 Naloxone:
A. Is a specific μ opioid receptor antagonist.
B. Reverses respiratory depression caused by pethidine.
C. May cause a rise in blood pressure.
D. Can cause pulmonary oedema.

4.48 Theme: Acid–base balance

Options:
A. Chronic bronchitis
B. Pain
C. Aspirin overdose
D. Potassium depletion
E. Renal tubular acidosis
F. Obstructive nephropathy

For each of the patients described below, select the single most likely diagnosis from the list of options above. Each option may be used once, more than once or not at all.

1. A 46-year-old male had a laryngectomy 24 h previously. He was extubated in theatre. He is an ex-smoker and gets breathless on moderate exercise. Routine arterial blood gases, taken on 24% oxygen, prior to his return to the ward were as follows: pH 7.52, PCO_2 5.3 kPa, PO_2 15.2 kPa, Hb saturation 100%, standard base excess (SBE) 7.9 meq/l.

2. A 24-year-old male is on ITU following a panproctocolectomy. He has the following blood gases: pH 7.55, PCO_2 3.24 kPa, PO_2 24.2 kPa, Hb saturation 100%, SBE 0.3 meq/l.

4.49 Theme: Hypotension

Options:
A. Pulmonary embolus
B. Tension pneumothorax
C. Severe dehydration
D. Sepsis
E. Acute myocardial infarction
F. Atrial fibrillation

For each of the patients described below, select the single most likely diagnosis from the list of options above. Each option may be used once, more than once or not at all.

1. A 28-year-old patient is being ventilated in the intensive care unit. He has been previously stable but suddenly his blood pressure falls to 70/40. On examination his pulse rate is 110 bpm, saturation 95% and CVP 6 cm H_2O.

2. A 46-year-old male has had a thoracotomy for carcinoma of the oesophagus 48 h previously. He was previously fit and well. The doctor is called when his blood pressure is noted to be 80/60. On examination, his heart rate is 115 bpm, saturation 96%, CVP 6 cm H_2O. ECG shows no abnormality of the ST segments.

3. Following an internal jugular CVP line insertion, a 50-year-old female becomes cyanosed with a saturation of 85%. Her heart rate is 105 bpm and her blood pressure is 90/55. CVP is 12 cm H_2O. Examination of her chest reveals bilateral air entry.

4.50 Theme: Urine output

Options:
A. Frusemide 1 mg/kg
B. Dobutamine 5–20 µg/kg
C. Fluid resuscitation
D. Central line
E. Haemodiafiltration

For each of the patients described below, select the single most appropriate therapy from the list of options above. Each option may be used once, more than once or not at all.

1. A patient weighing 60 kg is in the ITU following a thoracotomy 24 h previously. His condition is stable but his urine output has only been 100 ml over the last 6 h. On examination, his pulse rate is 98 bpm and his blood pressure is 95/50.

2. A 55-year-old man is admitted to ITU following a road traffic accident where he was the driver of the vehicle involved. Several hours after admission his urine output is only 15 ml/h despite aggressive fluid resuscitation. His CVP is 15 cm H_2O.

4.51 Theme: Cardiac drugs

Options:
A. Adrenaline
B. Ephedrine
C. Noradrenaline
D. GTN
E. Dobutamine

For each of the patients described below, select the single most likely therapy from the list of options above. Each option may be used once, more than once or not at all.

1. A 36-year-old female is admitted to ITU from casualty. On examination she has a pulse rate of 120 bpm, blood pressure of 70/50 and her systemic vascular resistance (SVR) is measured at 300 dyn s cm^{-5}.

2. A 56-year-old male is admitted to ITU following a cardiac arrest. On examination his heart rate is 90 bpm with a blood pressure of 78/60. His chest X-ray shows bilateral hilar shadowing.

3. A 60-year-old female is admitted to ITU following a cardiac arrest. On examination her heart rate is 80 bpm, blood pressure 130/90 and her chest X-ray shows upper lode diversion.

CORE MODULE **5**

Neoplasia, the breast, and techniques and outcome of surgery

NEOPLASIA

5.1 The following cancers have shown an increase in mortality over the last 60 years:
A. Lung.
B. Stomach.
C. Uterine.
D. Pancreatic.
E. Breast.

5.2 The following factors increase the risk of developing gastric cancer:
A. Male sex.
B. High socio-economic group.
C. Japanese ethnicity.
D. A diet high in vegetables and fruits.
E. A low salt intake.
F. Family history.
G. Blood group O.
H. A diet low in nitrates.

5.3 ⋆ The following are true of colorectal cancer:
A. There is an association with high red meat consumption.
B. There is an association with low intake of saturated fatty acids.
C. There is an association with low dietary fibre.
D. Fifty per cent of tumours arise in the sigmoid colon.
E. Patients with familial adenosis polyposis will usually present before the age of 40.
F. Tumours arising in patients with the hereditary non-polyposis colorectal cancer (HNPCC) gene are usually left sided.

5.4 ˙ Malignant melanoma:
A. Is associated with ionizing radiation.
B. Is more commonly seen on the trunks of women.
C. Occurs more commonly near the Equator.
D. Has a low incidence in peoples with pigmented skin.
E. Is associated with the dysplastic naevus syndrome.

5.5 ⁴ Peutz–Jeghers syndrome:
A. Is an inherited autosomal recessive condition.
B. Produces adenomatous polyps in the small intestine.
C. Is associated with circumoral pigmentation.
D. Is a predisposing factor in intussusception.
E. May present as a gastrointestinal bleed in childhood.
F. Is a premalignant condition.

5.6 ˀ With relation to benign and malignant tumours:
A. Malignant tumours have an expansile growth pattern.
B. Malignant tumours have a decrease in the nuclear/cytoplasmic ratio.
C. Malignant tumours show nuclear pleomorphism.
D. Benign tumours have normal cell/cell relationships.
E. Benign tumours show an increase in mitotic rate.

5.7 ˀ Adenomas:
A. Arise from columnar epithelium.
B. Do not have a capsule.
C. Will compress normal tissue around the lesion.
D. May have a cystic cut surface.
E. May be polyploid.

5.8 • **The following statements concerning the molecular basis of cancer are correct:**
   A. K-ras is a nuclear transcription factor.
   B. K-ras is mutated in 60–70% of colorectal cancers.
   C. Angiogenesis is inhibited by TNF (tumour necrosis factor) alpha.
   D. Metalloproteinases are implicated in metastasis.
   E. Cadherin loss promotes tumour invasion.

5.9 • **With respect to characteristics of malignancy:**
   A. A sessile lesion is more likely to be benign.
   B. A polypoid lesion is more likely to be malignant.
   C. A fungating lesion is more likely to be malignant.
   D. An ulcerated lesion is more likely to be benign.
   E. A papillary lesion is more likely to be benign.

5.10 **The following statements about lung cancer are correct:**
   A. It is increasing in incidence in men.
   B. It is associated with asbestos workers.
   C. Screening programmes have been ineffective.
   D. Ten per cent are incidental findings on chest radiographs.
   E. It may produce hyponatraemia.

5.11 **Oat cell (small cell) carcinomas of the lung:**
   A. Are usually amenable to surgery.
   B. Have a poorer survival rate than non-small cell tumours.
   C. Respond to chemotherapy.
   D. Are associated with reduced serum cortisol.
   E. Are usually disseminated at diagnosis.

5.12 **In colorectal cancers:**
   A. Approximately 5% of patients will have occult liver metastases at the time of diagnosis.
   B. Approximately 3% of patients will have a synchronous tumour on diagnosis of the primary.
   C. Carcinoma of the left colon classically presents with anaemia.
   D. Obstruction is more common in right than left sided tumours.
   E. Faecal occult blood testing has been shown to be a useful screening tool.

5.13 Renal cell cancer:
    A. Is more common in coffee drinkers.
    B. Is associated with cerebral angiomas.
    C. Usually spreads via the lymphatics.
    D. Commonly metastasizes to the lungs.
    E. Is more common in women.

5.14 Symptoms and signs associated with the presentation of renal cell cancers include:
    A. Fever.
    B. Deranged liver function tests.
    C. Hypocalcaemia.
    D. A right sided varicocoele.
    E. Hypoglycaemia.

5.15 The following statements concerning tumour markers are correct:
    A. CA l53 is a cytokeratin marker.
    B. CA 153 is associated with poorer prognosis in breast cancer if raised preoperatively.
    C. CA l53 is not useful in the early detection of breast cancer relapse.
    D. Neuron specific enolas are raised in advanced small cell lung cancers.
    E. Urinary VMMA is raised in carcinoid tumours.

5.16 The following statements about the molecular basis of cancer are correct:
    A. The p53 gene is found on chromosome 13.
    B. The retinoblastoma gene (Rb) is dominantly inherited.
    C. An oncogene is a normal component of cellular molecular physiology.
    D. P53 is found in small amounts in normal cells.
    E. C-erb B2 is a normal growth factor receptor.

5.17 In malignant melanoma:
  A. Breslow's thickness is a better prognostic indicator than Clark's levels.
  B. Men are more commonly affected.
  C. Ten per cent arise in a pre-existing naevus.
  D. Sites other than the skin can be affected.
  E. The most common type is nodular.
  F. A superficial spreading type is seen in uncovered areas.
  G. If thicker than 1 cm should be excised with a margin of 1 cm.

5.18 Hodgkin's disease:
  A. Accounts for 1% of newly diagnosed cancers.
  B. Has a unimodal age distribution.
  C. Is more common in firstborn children.
  D. Commonly presents with lymphadenopathy below the diaphragm.
  E. Patients have systemic 'B' symptoms in 70% of cases.
  F. Produces pain after alcohol ingestion.
  G. May have an extranodal site at presentation.
  H. Should be staged by computerized tomography of chest and abdomen.

5.19 In non-Hodgkin's lymphoma:
  A. Serum lactate dehydrogenase is a prognostic factor.
  B. Intrathoracic disease is less common than in Hodgkin's lymphoma.
  C. Few patients have bone marrow involvement.
  D. Renal failure is a recognized complication of treatment.
  E. The small intestine is the most common extranodal site of presentation.

5.20 Primary gastrointestinal lymphoma:
  A. Is usually of non-Hodgkin's type.
  B. Is usually of low grade.
  C. Is seen as a complication of coeliac disease.
  D. Rarely presents with perforation in the small intestine.
  E. In the small bowel is more common in the elderly.

5.21 Complications of radiotherapy include:
  A. An altered sense of taste.
  B. Constipation.
  C. Photosensitivity.
  D. Lumbar paraesthesia.
  E. Neutropenia.
  F. Lymphoedema.
  G. Ischaemic heart disease.

5.22 In radiotherapy:
  A. Iridium wires produce gamma rays.
  B. Electrons have greater tissue penetration than gamma rays.
  C. DNA damage occurs via an oxygen-dependent mechanism.
  D. Apoptosis can be initiated in normal cell lines.
  E. Most DNA damage is repaired within hours.

5.23 The following tumours are radiosensitive:
  A. Carcinoma of the pancreas.
  B. Testicular seminoma.
  C. Malignant melanoma.
  D. Malignant glioma.
  E. Hodgkin's lymphoma.

5.24 Radiotherapy:
  A. May be given preoperatively to improve local control after surgery.
  B. Preoperatively increases immediate surgical morbidity.
  C. Can be used to treat liver capsule pain from metastases.
  D. Effectively reduces pain from bone secondaries.
  E. Can be used to treat superior vena caval obstruction.

5.25 The following statements about chemotherapeutic agents are correct:
  A. Methotrexate is a cell phase dependent drug.
  B. Cyclophosphamide is an antitumour antibiotic.
  C. Vincristine is a vesicant drug.
  D. Interleukin 2 can be used to treat metastatic colonic cancer.
  E. Combination therapies reduce the development of drug resistance.

5.26 The following side effects are associated with these chemotherapeutic drugs:
A. Vomiting and cisplatinum.
B. Alopecia and 5-flourouracil.
C. Pulmonary fibrosis and vincristine.
D. Cardiotoxicity and doxorubicin.
E. Leukaemia and melphalan.

5.27 In relation to chemotherapy:
A. Choriocarcinoma is highly sensitive to chemotherapy agents.
B. Chemotherapy does not prolong survival in osteogenic sarcoma.
C. Carcinoma of the pancreas is poorly sensitive.
D. Chemotherapy may cure acute lymphoblastic leukaemia.
E. Chemotherapy has been shown to prolong survival in malignant melanoma.

5.28 The following statements regarding hormone sensitive tumours are correct:
A. If a breast tumour is oestrogen receptor positive there is a 100% response to hormone manipulation.
B. Oophorectomy is useful in post-menopausal breast cancer patients.
C. Tamoxifen is an oestrogen antagonist.
D. Cyproterone acetate may cause gynaecomastia.
E. Gonadotrophin releasing hormone analogues are useful in breast cancer.

5.29 The following statements concerning tumour markers are correct:
A. CEA (carcinoma embryonic antigen) is raised in 5% Dukes' B colorectal tumours.
B. CA 125 is found in normal pleural tissue.
C. PSA (prostatic specific antigen) is specific for prostate cancer.
D. AFP (alpha fetoprotein) can be used to screen populations at high risk of hepatocellular carcinoma.
E. CA 153 is a marker of pancreatic cancer.
F. CA 125 can be used to screen for carcinoma of the ovary.

5.30 Theme: Physical and chemical carcinogens

Options:
A. Aniline dyes
B. Polyvinyl chloride
C. Asbestos
D. Ultraviolet radiation
E. Ionizing radiation
F. Chromium
G. Benzene
H. Nickel

For each of the malignancies described below, select the single carcinogen most often associated with it from the list of options above. Each option may be used once, more than once or not at all.

1. Mesothelioma.

2. Thyroid cancer.

3. Cancers of the nasal cavity.

4. Transitional cell carcinoma of the urinary tract.

5. Hepatocellular carcinoma.

5.31 Theme: Renal tumours

Options:
A. Renal cell carcinoma
B. Angiomyolipoma
C. Transitional cell cancer
D. Juxtaglomerular tumour
E. Oncocytoma
F. Lipoma
G. Haemangiopericytoma

For each of the patients described below, select the single most likely diagnosis from the list of options above. Each option may be used once, more than once or not at all.

1. A 46-year-old man with a portwine stain on his face since birth and a history of epilepsy presents with a mass in his right loin. A CT scan showed a large tumour with both hypo- and hyperdense areas with no obvious invasion into the renal vein.

2. A 52-year-old man with recurrent bouts of hypoglycaemia and hypertension associated with hypernatraemia was found on abdominal imaging to have a l cm tumour in the right renal cortex

3. A 70-year-old man presents with a low grade fever, anaemia, lethargy and muscle fatigue. Examination reveals a large mass in the right loin and there is +++ for blood on urine dipstix.

5.32 Theme: Tumour, node, metastasis staging (TNM)

Options:
A. T2 N1 MO
B. T2 N2 MO
C. T2 NI MI
D. T4 N3 MO
E. T4 N1 MO

For each of the patients described below, select the single most likely stage from the list of options above. Each option may be used once, more than once or not at all.

1. A 36-year-old women who is breast feeding has noticed that her right breast is red, swollen and hard. She has not responded to a course of antibiotics given by her GP. At breast clinic triple assessment reveals an 8 cm carcinoma centrally with some mobile nodes in the ipsilateral axilia.

2. A 64-year-old women presents to breast clinic having ignored a lump of 3 cm in her left upper outer quadrant with skin fixation. There are palpable nodes in the left axilia and supraclavicular fossa.

3. A 53-year-old woman presents to breast clinic with a 2.5 cm tumour in the right upper inner quadrant. Hard fixed matted nodes are found in the right axilla.

5.33 Theme: Palliative treatments

Options:
A. Radiotherapy
B. Subcutaneous opiate infusion
C. Dexamethasone
D. Coeliac plexus block
E. Tricyclic antidepressants
F. Surgical fixation

For each of the patients described below, select the single most appropriate treatment from the list of options above. Each option may be used once, more than once or not at all.

1. A 38-year-old woman with known metastatic breast cancer and a young family presents with severe right hip pain. A plain X-ray shows erosion of 80% of the cortex of the upper femur and a bone scan also shows metastases in the ribs.

2. A 64-year-old man who had an anterior resection for a Dukes' C carcinoma 18 months previously presents early to outpatient follow up with severe right upper quadrant pain of one week's duration that did not respond to moderate analgesics. Examination reveals a knobbly liver 2 cm below the costal margin.

3. A 78-year-old man presents with severe epigastric pain radiating to the back and jaundice. An ultrasound scan showed a 5 cm mass in the head of the pancreas. A biliary stent was inserted at ERCP. The pain failed to resolve on standard analgesics.

THE BREAST

5.34 The female breast:
  A. Is derived from the mesodermal layer of the embryo.
  B. Represents a modified sweat gland.
  C. Overlies the 2nd to 6th ribs.
  D. Is supplied by branches of the internal thoracic artery.
  E. Responds to insulin levels during pregnancy.

5.35 Structures identified during axillary clearance include:
  A. The long thoracic nerve.
  B. The subclavian vein.
  C. The intercostobrachial nerve.
  D. The thoracodorsal trunk.
  E. The medial pectoral nerve.

5.36 Specific complications of surgical axillary dissection include:
  A. Upper limb lymphoedema.
  B. Brachial plexus traction neuropraxia.
  C. Weakness over the deltoid muscle.
  D. Weakness of shoulder elevation.
  E. 'Winging' of the scapula.

5.37 Breast mammography:
  A. Is most helpful in women under 50.
  B. Should be carried out annually in women over 50 with a family history of breast cancer.
  C. Sensitivity is improved using a breast coil.
  D. Specificity is improved by use of contrast.
  E. Does not show breast cysts.

5.38 The following conditions may cause nipple discharge:
  A. Posterior pituitary tumours.
  B. Mondor's disease.
  C. Intraductal papilloma.
  D. Phylloides tumour.
  E. Duct ectasia.

5.39 Cyclical mastalgia:
  A. Is commonly associated with lobular breast cancer.
  B. Is relieved by HRT.
  C. Is effectively relieved by surgical excision.
  D. Often responds to treatment with evening primrose oil.
  E. Is treated by danazol in severe cases.

5.40 Gynaecomastia is associated with:
  A. Spironolactone.
  B. Digoxin.
  C. Turner syndrome.
  D. Anabolic steroids.
  E. Bronchial carcinoma.

5.41 Tamoxifen:
  A. Is not indicated in oestrogen receptor positive tumours.
  B. Is discontinued after two years.
  C. Increases the risk of stroke.
  D. Increases the risk of ovarian cancer.
  E. Increases the risk of endometrial cancer.

5.42 The following syndromes are associated with an increased risk of breast cancer:
  A. Li–Fraumeni.
  B. Poland.
  C. AIDS.
  D. Von Hippel–Lindau.
  E. Dandy–Walker.

5.43 The following factors are associated with increased risk of breast cancer:
  A. Prolonged HRT (hormone replacement therapy).
  B. Early menopause.
  C. Nulliparity.
  D. Previous chest wall irradiation.
  E. Obesity.

5.44 Locally advanced breast cancer is defined if:
A. The tumour is greater than 3 cm diameter.
B. There is skin oedema (*peau d'orange*).
C. Fixed axillary nodes are palpable.
D. There is nipple retraction.
E. Widespread breast inflammation can be seen.

5.45 Fine needle aspiration cytology (FNAC):
A. Is only performed on post-menopausal women.
B. Normally requires preinfiltration with local anaesthetic.
C. Should be repeated if a C2 result is given.
D. Usually has a sensitivity of over 90%.
E. Has a high false positive rate.

5.46 The following are associated with poor prognosis in breast cancer:
A. The tumour is strongly positive for oestrogen receptors.
B. Grade III tumour (Bloom and Richardson classification).
C. Medullary carcinoma.
D. Expression of Ki 67 nuclear antigen.
E. Tumours less than 0.5 cm diameter.

5.47 Breast conservation surgery is usually contraindicated if:
A. Axillary nodes are palpable.
B. The patient refuses radiotherapy.
C. There is extensive DCIS.
D. The tumour is lobular carcinoma.
E. Tumour size is greater than 4 cm.

5.48 In level III dissection of the axilla:
A. The axillary vein marks the upper limit of the surgery.
B. The intercostobrachial nerve is sometimes sacrificed.
C. The pectoralis minor muscle is removed.
D. The indications include extensive DCIS.
E. Adjuvant radiotherapy is required if nodes are involved.

5.49 Metastatic disease from breast cancer:
    A. Has a mean survival rate of six months.
    B. May present as breathlessness.
    C. Forms mainly lytic bone lesions.
    D. Rarely responds to primary hormonal treatment alone.
    E. Is more common in mucinous tumours.

5.50 Ductal carcinoma in situ (DCIS):
    A. Shows up as calcification on mammograms.
    B. Should be treated with primary chemotherapy.
    C. Rarely becomes invasive if left untreated.
    D. May occur in association with Paget's disease of the nipple.
    E. Is usually bilateral.

5.51 Fibroadenomas:
    A. Are composed of fibrous and glandular tissue.
    B. Are more common in post-menopausal women.
    C. Tend to undergo malignant transformation if left untreated.
    D. Typically vary in size during the menstrual cycle.
    E. Can be characterized on ultrasound.

5.52 Benign mammary dysplasia:
    A. Is more common in post-menopausal women.
    B. Commonly presents with mastalgia.
    C. May result in multiple cyst formation.
    D. Is stimulated by HRT.
    E. Is also known as fibroadenosis.

5.53 Male breast cancer:
    A. Accounts for less than 2% of all cases of breast cancer.
    B. Has a higher incidence of lobular-type cancer than in females.
    C. Does not have a familial tendency.
    D. Has an older median age of presentation than in females.
    E. Tumours rarely express oestrogen or progesterone receptors.

5.54 The national screening programme for breast cancer:
   A. Invites women aged 55–65 years for screening.
   B. Is available only for women who have first-degree relatives with breast cancer.
   C. Uses imaging with mammograms and ultrasound.
   D. Routinely recalls women after three years.
   E. Is not available for younger women.

5.55 The following tests are routinely done in staging newly diagnosed breast cancer:
   A. Liver function tests.
   B. Full blood count.
   C. Chest radiograph.
   D. CT of the head.
   E. Bone scan.

5.56 Follow up of treated breast cancer routinely involves:
   A. Regular clinical examination.
   B. Annual bone scan.
   C. Annual mammography.
   D. Annual serum CA 153 level.
   E. Annual serum carcinoembryonic antigen (CEA) level.

5.57 Chemotherapy for breast cancer:
   A. Is only indicated if nodes are involved.
   B. Normally requires a six month course.
   C. Commonly uses CMF (cyclophosphamide, methotrexate, 5FU).
   D. Has greatest benefit in premenopausal women.
   E. Has no role in palliation of the disease.

5.58 Breast reconstruction using a latissimus dorsi flap:
   A. Is not recommended at the time of initial surgery.
   B. Utilizes the thoracodorsal pedicle.
   C. Requires use of the latissimus dorsi muscle with or without overlying skin.
   D. Can be used in conjunction with a tissue expander.
   E. Normally requires a microvascular anastomosis.

5.59 Phylloides tumour of the breast:
A. Most commonly occurs in patients aged over 70 years.
B. Is usually very locally aggressive.
C. Responds to radiotherapy.
D. Is associated with Paget's disease of the nipple.
E. May resemble sarcoma histologically.

5.60 Paget's disease of the nipple:
A. May be initially confused with eczema.
B. Is frequently bilateral.
C. Rarely indicates underlying malignancy in the absence of a lump.
D. Can be treated with local radiotherapy.
E. Can result from prolonged lactation.

5.61 In the TNM staging classification:
A. T4 indicates a tumour size greater than 5 cm in diameter.
B. T1 indicates a tumour less than 2 cm in diameter.
C. MX indicates metastatic disease is present.
D. *Peau d'orange* is classified as TIS.
E. N2 indicates fixed homolateral axillary nodes.

5.62 The following statements concerning invasive breast cancer are correct:
A. Ductal type is the most common.
B. Mucinous type tends to be more aggressive.
C. Lobular type is more commonly bilateral.
D. Tubular type tends to be well differentiated.
E. Medullary type is characterized by lymphocytic infiltration.

5.63 Fat necrosis of the breast:
A. Often follows trauma.
B. Is more common in post-menopausal women.
C. May be associated with skin inflammation.
D. Can present as a hard lump.
E. Has a small risk of malignant transformation.

5.64 The following statements concerning the BRCA 1 gene are correct:

A. It is found on the long arm of chromosome 17.
B. It is implicated in the majority of all breast cancers.
C. Mutation results in the Li–Fraumeni syndrome.
D. Mutation gives rise to high incidence of premenopausal breast cancer.
E. It is also associated with increased risk of ovarian cancer.

5.65 Carcinoma of the breast:

A. Has a higher incidence in the Far East.
B. Is more common in the Ashkenazi Jewish population.
C. Occurs mainly in high-risk families.
D. Is associated with cervical cancer.
E. Is associated with excessive radiation exposure.

5.66 Theme: First-line management plan

Options:
A. Outpatient follow up only
B. Primary chemotherapy
C. Lumpectomy
D. Segmental mastectomy + radiotherapy, axillary clearance
E. Total mastectomy +/– reconstruction
F. Total mastectomy, axillary clearance
G. Primary radiotherapy
H. Primary hormonal treatment (tamoxifen 20 mg/day).

For each of the patients described below, select the single most appropriate first-line treatment from the list of options above. Each option may be used once, more than once or not at all.

1. An 88-year-old woman presents with a firm 2.5 cm lump in the right lower breast. FNAC shows C5 with oestrogen receptor positive.

2. A 37-year-old woman, presents with 4 cm lump in left axillary tail. Nodes palpable in the axilla. Mammography and FNAC confirm invasive ductal carcinoma.

3. A 51-year-old female with widespread microcalcification noted throughout the breast on screening mammography. FNAC C1. Multiple core biopsy shows DCIS but no invasive disease.

4. A 56-year-old woman with a positive family history of breast cancer. Lump in left lateral breast. Mammogram and ultrasound suggestive of fibroadenoma. FNAC is C2.

5. A 55-year-old man, who is a heavy drinker, presents with a painful swollen right breast. US and FNAC within normal limits. Liver function tests abnormal.

6. A 37-year-old female presents with cyclical pain. Nodular breasts but no discrete lump. US and mammogram normal.

7. A 66-year-old female with a swollen, red right nipple. No lump palpable. Nipple biopsy suggests Paget's disease.

8. A 53-year-old woman with a 2 cm diameter lump in right axillary tail. FNA C5. Mammogram confirms carcinoma.

TECHNIQUES AND OUTCOME OF SURGERY

5.67 Informed consent for surgical procedures:
A. Must be a signed document using a specially printed consent form.
B. Should explain the nature of the condition and the prognosis of the proposed treatment.
C. Should include the common and uncommon side effects of anaesthesia.
D. Should include an explanation of alternative treatments.
E. Does not preclude the patient from having the right to withdraw consent to treatment at any time.

5.68 The following statements concerning surgical procedures are correct:
A. Treatment of patients without their consent constitutes assault and battery.
B. Informed consent involves telling patients about every possible complication.
C. The parents or guardians of minors under the age of 16 years should give consent for surgical procedures.
D. The Bolam principle relates to the treatment of patients who are unable to give their consent.

5.69 In palliative care:
A. Nausea and vomiting should not be treated.
B. Dry mouth may be caused by analgesics.
C. Hyoscine can reduce secretions from the trachea and bronchi.
D. Constipation is rarely relieved by laxatives.
E. Midazolam is contraindicated as a sedative.

5.70 The following statements about analgesia in palliative care are correct:
- A. NSAIDs are not useful as analgesics.
- B. The maximum dose of morphine is 10 mg every four hours.
- C. Diamorphine can only be given subcutaneously.
- D. Modified-release morphine preparations may be administered once daily.
- E. Analgesics given transdermally via patches are not effective.

5.71 Regarding analgesia in palliative care:
- A. Opioids may cause nausea and vomiting.
- B. Constipation is not caused by opioids.
- C. Nerve pain may be reduced by carbamazepine.
- D. Corticosteroids can reduce tumour oedema and swelling, thus reducing pain.
- E. Morphine may cause dry mouth.

5.72 In managing palliative care:
- A. Nerve blocks can relieve localized pain.
- B. TENS is not useful for pain relief.
- C. Diazepam can be given for muscle pain.
- D. Syringe drivers can be used to deliver intramuscular diamorphine.
- E. Only analgesics can be delivered via syringe drivers.

5.73 The following are types of audit:
- A. Structure.
- B. Process.
- C. Outcome.
- D. Manpower.
- E. Treatment.

5.74 Audit of outcome includes:
- A. Morbidity.
- B. Mortality.
- C. Symptom relief.
- D. Patient satisfaction.
- E. Quality of life.
- F. Length of hospital stay.

5.75 Clinical audit includes:
A. Observation of current practice.
B. Comparison of current practice with a set standard.
C. Changes to current practice which close the 'audit loop'.
D. Observation of new practice and comparison with old practice.
E. Systematic critical analysis of the quality of medical care.

5.76 The following statements are true:
A. Audit seeks to define best practice and determines what constitutes good care.
B. Research determines if good care is being practised.
C. Clinical trials compare the effect and value of intervention against controls.
D. Medical audit is assessment of patient care provided by doctors.
E. Clinical audit assess the total care of the patient by all healthcare professionals.

Perioperative management (I)

1.1 **A.** False
B. False
C. True
D. True
E. True

Wound healing by secondary intention takes place when the wound breaks apart, when the wound edges are not brought together, and when there is irreparable skin loss. When the wound becomes infected and is laid open, healing is also by secondary intention. If the edges are opposed, for example in a sutured wound, the healing is by primary intention. Healing in this way is much slower compared with healing by first intention.

1.2 **A.** False
B. True
C. False
D. True
E. True

Acute metabolic acidosis is the main feature of total body hypoxia as seen in cardiac arrest. It is the result of inadequate tissue perfusion, and the failure of aerobic pathways of energy supply. It can result from prolonged cross clamping of the aorta during aneurysm repair and is present when the whole body has been underperfused for an hour or more.

1.3   **A.** False
      B. True
      C. False
      D. True
      E. True

Early septic shock postoperatively in surgical patients does require early dialysis if there is acute renal failure. It may present with warm hypotension which may progress to cold hypotension. Cold hypotension is associated with a high mortality of 70%. It is also part of the SIRS (systemic immune response syndrome) which is mediated by the release of nitric oxide. Septic shock is commonly of the hyperdynamic type, that is, with raised cardiac output and reduced peripheral resistance.

1.4   **A.** True
      B. False
      C. False
      D. False
      E. False

At operation, the open wound is at risk of contamination from operating room personnel. Positive pressure filtered ventilation of the operating theatre prevents bacteria from gaining entry with the air. Modern ultraclean ventilation and the use of fine filters only reduces the rate of wound infection twofold. The patient's own skin is a source of infection. The use of a plastic adhesive film (Opsite), through which the incision is made, may reduce but does not prevent contamination.

1.5 A. False
   B. True
   C. False
   D. False
   E. True

Necrotizing fasciitis is caused by mixture of Staphylococci and Streptococci including anaerobic and microaerophilic cocci, therefore antibiotic therapy and hyperbaric oxygen do limit the spread of infection. The skin initially appears normal. Bold and wide surgical excision of the necrotic fascia, skin and muscle should be carried out immediately without delay. This condition is very common with i.v. drug abuse. High doses of benzylpenicillin intravenously are indicated.

1.6 A. False
   B. True
   C. True
   D. False
   E. True

Early wound infection and inflammation are characterized by an increase in blood flow and vascular permeability in the affected area, hence the erythema which is seen. Phagocytes infiltrate locally to phagocytose any microbes and damaged tissue. It is rarely associated with deep-seated abscess collections. The inflammatory response is dependent on the burden of tissue injury, that is, the greater the volume of tissue affected, the greater the inflammatory response.

1.7 **A.** False
  B. False
  C. True
  D. False
  E. True

In the management of surgical wound infections, surgical debridement of damaged, necrotic tissue and the drainage of pus collections are essential. Excess retraction of small wounds can affect the infection rate. Complete haemostasis is essential as haematomas are a good culture medium for bacteria. The presence of a deadspace during wound closure delays wound healing, as the space may be occupied by haematoma or seroma. The wound should be closed with layer-to-layer approximation with no tension as this causes ischaemia of the tissues.

1.8 **A.** True
  B. True
  C. False
  D. True
  E. False

A prolonged period of therapy with parenteral antibiotics is indicated in progression of infection despite adequate drainage, septicaemia and in immunocompromised patients. Systemic antibiotics are rarely indicated for the treatment of uncomplicated wound abscesses which can be surgically drained. A short-term antibiotic prophylactic cover for anaerobic organisms is usually adequate in normal colonic surgery.

1.9 **A.** True
    B. True
    C. True
    D. True
    E. True

Hypoalbuminaemia is associated with delayed wound healing and immune deficiency. Morbid obesity is associated with high risks of wound and other infections, for example in the chest. Concurrent sepsis reduces patients' immunity and they are therefore more vulnerable to further infections. Location and duration of operation can increase risks of contamination and infection; for example in emergency colonic surgery without bowel preparation. The long-term use of prophylactic antibiotics does result in an increased risk of infection especially with resistant organisms.

1.10 A. False
    B. True
    C. False
    D. True
    E. True

Mass muscle closure with non-absorbable sutures or absorbable sutures with a long half-life is recommended. Wound healing by secondary intention in the presence of major intra-abdominal sepsis remains a safe option. A laparostomy is when the abdomen is left open and the wound allowed to granulate. Any intra-abdominal collections will drain out of the wound. Closure with a continuous suture four times as long as the incision is neccessary. The risk of wound infection and hence wound breakdown is reduced with antibiotic prophylaxis at induction. Preoperative correction of malnutrition improves wound healing and reduces the risk of dehiscence.

1.11 A. True
B. False
C. False
D. False
E. False

Meticulous surgical techniques including gentle tissue handling and avoidance of spillage from the bowel can improve wound healing. Skin shaving 24–48 h before surgery increases the risk of infection by causing tiny skin abrasions. Incising the skin along the lines of Langer does not affect healing except by cosmetic result. Local injection of steroids delays wound healing. The use of prophylactic antibiotics for five days postoperatively has no affect on wound healing when compared to the administration of just two postoperative doses.

1.12 A. True
B. False
C. False
D. True
E. True
F. True

The APACHE II scoring system is used to compare treatment regimens. It uses disease-specific weighting factors to calculate mortality. The Glasgow Coma Scale forms part of the APACHE II score. Chronic conditions affecting the liver, cardiovascular and pulmonary function are all considered in the APACHE II score and in the prediction of mortality. A score above 21 correlates with a mortality risk of 50%. An acute physiology score and a chronic health evaluation are the two integrated parts of the APACHE II system.

1.13 A. True
  B. True
  C. True
  D. False
  E. True

Adverse effects of perioperative blood transfusion include risk of CMV infection and risk of Hepatitis B and C infections, even though the blood is screened for these and other infections including HIV. There is a risk of iron overload and of alloimmunization, especially in patients with haemoglobinopathy who have had numerous transfusions. Transfusion is associated with graft-versus-host disease where the WBCs in the donor blood recognize the recipient antigens as foreign and react to them.

1.14 A. True
  B. True
  C. False
  D. True
  E. False
  F. True

In synergistic gangrene, the initial cellulitis is followed by progressive gangrenous ulceration. By definition, it is the synergistic action of aerobic haemolytic Staphylococci and microaerophilic non-haemolytic Streptococci. Meleney's burrowing ulcers are caused by haemolytic microaerophilic Streptococci. The skin necrosis characteristically has a metallic sheen. In gas gangrene it is the release of powerful exotoxins by Clostridia that cause local tissue necrosis. The diagnosis is based on typical clinical findings and the presence of large Gram-positive rods in the wound fluid.

1.15 A. False
B. True
C. True
D. True
E. True
F. False

In surgical infections, contamination can occur follow penetrating and blunt abdominal trauma. Secondary peritonitis is common when the laparotomy for traumatic intestinal rupture is performed 24 h or more after the injury. Hepatic capsulitis with pelvic infection (Curtis–Fitz–Hugh syndrome) may mimic cholecystitis. It is caused by *Chlamydia trachomatis* and is treated with tetracycline. Obligate anaerobes are found in more than 50% of liver abscesses. A localized paracolic diverticular abscess can be drained percutaneously under ultrasound or CT guidance, especially in the elderly and unfit patients. Pancreatitis begins as a chemical inflammation but most of the fatalities are caused by infections.

1.16 A. True
B. False
C. True
D. False
E. False
F. False

In postoperative wound infections with collections reopening the wound and evacuating the pus is the optimal treatment. The diagnosis is mainly clinical. Preoperative shaving increases the incidence of wound infection and is time related. Shaving immediately preoperatively causes less infection than shaving of the area the day before operation. Antibiotic prophylaxis should be given at the time of induction of anaesthesia followed by further doses postoperatively. The signs of superficial infection are local erythema, pain and induration, that is, local inflammatory response. The nutritional status of the patient greatly affects healing and the incidence of wound infection is greater in malnourished patients with, for example, hypoalbuminaemia.

1.17 A. False
  B. True
  C. True
  D. True
  E. True

Adequate laminar flow system in the operating theatres is essential to direct contaminated air away from the operative field. Interrupted vertical mattress sutures are used where the skin edges may not be approximated accurately because of tissue laxity.

Modern electrocautery machines employ a rheostat to vary the output current to achieve coagulation and haemostasis. The bipolar diathermy machine uses a low current at very high frequency and high voltage passing through the patient's tissue using two electrodes to complete the circuit. Bipolar diathermy should be used if the patient has a pacemaker in place so that the current arcs across the two tips of the diathermy instrument and does not have to travel through the patient to the diathermy plate, which may cause the pacemaker to malfunction.

1.18 A. False
  B. False
  C. False
  D. True
  E. True

In patients with chronic respiratory symptoms, and in patients with cardiomyopathy with a normal chest X-ray six months earlier, a preoperative chest X-ray is not required if symptoms are stable and the previous X-ray is satisfactory. A 50-year-old patient undergoing routine abdominal operation is fit and healthy and there is no indication for X-ray. In a 30-year-old patient with malignancy, it may detect occult metastatic disease. In a 25-year-old patient who is a recent immigrant, chest X-ray is required as pulmonary TB or other respiratory infections cannot be ruled out.

1.19 A. False
  B. False
  C. True
  D. False
  E. False

Heparin anticoagulation is reversed by the cessation of heparin infusion or administration of protamine. Vitamin K can be used to help reverse the effects of warfarin. Heparin has longer action when administered subcutaneously as the absorption into the system is slower. Thrombocytopenia is a recognized side effect. Heparin is cleared from the body mainly by hepatic metabolism. Low molecular weight heparin should be used intravenously to treat iliac vein thrombosis but can be used subcutaneously for the treatment of deep femoral and calf vein thromboses.

1.20 A. False
  B. True
  C. True
  D. False
  E. False

For a 70-year-old male smoker prior to total gastrectomy, liver function can be normal even with advanced hepatic metastases. Chest X-ray can be used as a preoperative screening for respiratory and cardiac pathology. Laparoscopy can be used for preoperative staging whilst a barium swallow is not. Gastroscopy provides direct visualization of disease and biopsy for histology, but is not useful for staging unless combined with endoluminal ultrasound.

1.21 A. False
    B. True
    C. True
    D. True
    E. True

Obesity predisposes to deep venous thrombosis whether a patient has surgery or not. Laparoscopic surgery is often easier for patients in the postoperative period as the respiratory function is better because of decreased wound pain, and they can be mobilized early; for the surgeons, the procedure may be technically easier. Increased tendency to hypertension, diabetes and arthritis are frequent problems with morbid obesity. Increased incidence of wound haematoma, dehiscence and infection are all associated with deep subcutaneous cavities.

1.22 A. True
    B. True
    C. True
    D. False
    E. True
    F. False

Thyroid cancer should be treated by subtotal thyroidectomy with TSH suppression using thyroxine supplements. [131]I therapy has no role to play in preoperative management but may be used postoperatively for the treatment of metastases, local recurrence or residual tumour. Treatment with high doses of thyroxine is effective in suppressing TSH release and thus thyroid stimulation, and future recurrence. Chemotherapy is rarely effective in the treatment of recurrences. Block dissection of the lymph nodes in the neck has no effect on prognosis.

1.23 A. True
  B. True
  C. True
  D. True
  E. False

In patients with morbid obesity, epidural PCA is the recommended method of analgesia as the absorption of intramuscular and subcutaneous injections is very variable. Sitting up postoperatively reduces hypoventilation and hypoxia. The rate of anaesthetic and surgical complications is generally higher. Early mobilization is very important to avoid respiratory and venous complications. Thromboembolic deterrent stockings are very important postoperatively.

1.24 A. True
  B. False
  C. True
  D. False
  E. True

The first stage of tubular bone fracture healing starts with the fracture haematoma. Cell proliferation at the fracture site then occurs. They produce woven bone which is then transformed to lamellar bone by the osteoblasts. The callus at the site is more profuse in children. Bone remodelling in children after a fracture is so perfect that the site of the fracture eventually becomes indistinguishable in radiographs.

1.25 A. False
  B. True
  C. True
  D. True
  E. True

Needle-track seedlings in a patient with suspected primary carcinoma considered to be suitable for thoracotomy can happen, which can compromise the cure rate. FNA in suspected lung metastases can help to plan palliative treatment. In a primary lung mass suspected as a source of metastases elsewhere, FNA is used to confirm diagnosis prior to palliative treatment. In suspected localized infectious process, FNA can identify if empyema or if a localized abscess is present, and provide a specimen for culture. FNA can be adequate for the diagnosis of amyloidosis.

1.26 A. True
   B. False
   C. False
   D. False
   E. False

Acute osteomyelitis is common in children under the age of ten years. Positive blood cultures are very common, and help to identify the organism. Staphylococcal infection is the most common causative organism. A haematogenous source of the infection occurs in more than 25% of cases. High doses of systemic antibiotics are usually effective.

1.27 A. True
   B. True
   C. True
   D. True
   E. True
   F. True

Mycobacterium avium intracellulare is a common infection in AIDS patients. Enterocolitis may be caused by cytomegalovirus and *Salmonella typhi* in these patients. Kaposi's sarcoma is a common malignancy in AIDS. Acute and chronic perianal sepsis are frequently encountered, as is herpes simplex perianal chronic infection.

1.28 A. True
   B. True
   C. True
   D. True
   E. True
   F. True

Antithrombin III inhibits the formation of fibrin, and its deficiency results in hypercoagulability. Nephrotic syndrome causes hypoproteinaemia and sluggish circulation and also causes anti-thrombin III stimulation. Varicose veins cause sluggish venous circulation and predispose to DVT. Hypotensive anaesthesia is associated with sluggish circulation. Previous thrombophlebitis is associated with abnormalities in the vein wall. Cancer is associated with hypercoagulability.

1.29 A. False
B. False
C. True
D. False
E. False
F. True

The germination of tetanus spores in a wound is inhibited by oxygen and surgical debridement of devitalized tissue. It is accelerated by tissue trauma, the presence of foreign bodies, and by the injection of booster adsorbed toxoid and of booster antitoxin.

1.30 A. False
B. True
C. True
D. True
E. False

Clostridium tetani causes tetanus, and it produces a very powerful exotoxin which is neurotoxic. A characteristic feature of the spores is a terminal spore. It is an obligatory anaerobe and is motile.

1.31 A. True
B. True
C. True
D. True
E. True

Prophylactic antibiotics reduce the rate of infections in elective, 'clean' colorectal surgery. Although breast surgery is 'clean surgery', there is a high risk of infection of the prosthesis in breast reconstruction. Amputation is usually associated with vascular ischaemia and necrotic tissue, together with risks of gas gangrene and wound infection requiring antibiotic prophylaxis. Antibiotic prophylaxis reduces the risks of infective endocarditis and septicaemia in patients with heart valve abnormalities. Prophylactic antibiotics reduce the risk of infection in patients with a foreign body prostheses.

1.32 A. True
  B. False
  C. True
  D. True
  E. True

The immunocompromised include HIV-positive patients, patients who have received a blood transfusion of more than two units, are hypoxic or diabetic.

1.33 A. True
  B. True
  C. True
  D. True
  E. False
  F. True

Neoplasia delays wound healing, and is frequently associated with malnutrition. Adhesions to bony surfaces affect the contraction of the scar and neovascularization. Nephrotic syndrome is associated with hypoproteinaemia. Exposure to ionizing radiation reduces the healing rate by causing cell death. Vitamin C deficiency delays wound healing, whilst exposure to ultraviolet light improves it.

1.34 A. True
  B. False
  C. False
  D. True
  E. False
  F. True

Vasoconstriction and raised plasma levels of catecholamines are part of the ebb phase of the body's response to trauma and stress. The body's response to trauma includes increased glycogenolysis in the liver, decreased secretions of insulin, increased plasma levels of glycerol and serum fatty acids, a negative nitrogen balance, and increased gluconeogenesis in the liver to provide glucose to vital organs.

1.35 A. True
    B. False
    C. False
    D. False
    E. False

Local anaesthetic infiltration does reduce the requirement for opioid analgesics. Intramuscular opioid injections do not give adequate or reliable uptake for pain relief. Pethidine analgesic effects last for 3 h or less. Oral analgesia should be given *before* the pain is re-established. Patient-controlled analgesia is poorly delivered in most elderly patients.

1.36 A. False
    B. True
    C. False
    D. True
    E. True

Diclofenac is a non-steroidal antiinflammatory drug (NSAID). Suppository preparations can cause rectal ulceration in patients with inflammatory bowel disease. It is contraindicated in patients with asthma as it may cause bronchospasm – as can other NSAIDs. It is also contraindicated in patients with epigastric pain and melaena. A dose of 75 mg b.d. is useful in a patient with ureteric colic. As with most NSAIDs it can cause further renal impairment.

1.37 A. False
    B. True
    C. True
    D. True
    E. True

Acute visceral pain can be caused by distension of the hollow viscera, ischaemia, torsion or traction stress to the mesentery, and spasms of the smooth muscle of the hollow viscera. Cutting or burning of the hollow viscera causes somatic pain.

1.38 A. True
 B. True
 C. False
 D. False
 E. True

Visceral pain can be exacerbated by eating and movement, and can be referred to distant regions of the body supplied by the same somatic roots. A *small* number of afferent fibres usually represent *large* visceral areas. The pain is not sharply localized to specific visceral regions and is accompanied by powerful motor and autonomic reactions with increased sympathetic outflow.

1.39 A. False
 B. True
 C. True
 D. True
 E. False

The advantage of adding adrenaline to local anaesthetic is that the total dose can be greater because it slows the systemic absorption of local anaesthetic by causing vasoconstriction and hence also has a longer duration of action. There is then also less bleeding from the wound, but it has an adverse effect on healing in areas of poor tissue perfusion.

1.40 A. False
 B. False
 C. False
 D. True
 E. False
 F. False

The most likely diagnosis is ascending cholangitis. Pancreatitis does not usually present with symptoms of septicaemia. The most likely pathogenic causes of the sepsis are Gram-negative bacilli, Enterococci and anaerobes. Benzylpenicillin does not give good cover to anaerobes and is not the treatment of choice. An intravenous combination of gentamicin and metronidazole gives good cover. Prophylactic antibiotics therapy should prevent this complication of ERCP. An emergency repeat ERCP would exacerbate cholangitis and is therefore not recommended.

1.41 A. False
   B. False
   C. True
   D. True
   E. True

Subcutaneous heparin prior to an insertion of an epidural line increases the risk of bleeding complications as a result of epidural catheter insertion, and should be commenced postoperatively. Antibiotic prophylaxis should be administered at induction of anaesthesia and not together with the bowel preparation. Compartment pressure syndrome in the legs is a recognized complication of prolonged positioning of the legs in Lloyd-Davies or lithotomy. Intravenous fluids are given prior to surgery to correct dehydration and to ensure that the intravascular compartment is well filled prior to the expansion of the vascular spaces as a result of anaesthesia. Excess blood transfusion may impair the immune system in addition to the immunosuppression caused by malignant disease.

1.42 A. True
   B. True
   C. True
   D. True
   E. False

Pleural effusion in a postoperative surgical patient following abdominal surgery can result from pneumonia, which is a common cause, and congestive cardiac failure. Subdiaphragmatic abscess can cause sympathetic pleural effusion. Hypoalbuminaemia causes oedema and transudate effusion. Atelectasis does not cause effusion.

1.43 A. True
  B. False
  C. True
  D. True
  E. True
  F. True

Risk factors for developing abdominal incisional hernia include diabetes, anaemia and hypoalbuminaemia, all of which cause delayed wound healing. Previous abdominal surgery does not normally affect the healing. Morbid obesity increases risks of wound dehiscence because of pressure and tension on the wound. Intra-abdominal malignancy and an increase in intra-abdominal pressure are also associated with increased risks of wound dehiscence owing to poor healing and ischaemia respectively.

1.44 A. True
  B. False
  C. False
  D. False
  E. True

Pyrexia and sepsis following a low anterior resection indicates an anastomotic leak until proven otherwise. Pyrexia and sepsis two days after surgery is too early for DVT. It is also too early for chest infection, but such pyrexia can be caused by atelectasis. It is rarely indicative of subphrenic abscess. Pyrexia and sepsis following elective abdominal surgery calls for careful examination of the wound and rectal examination to detect any wound infection or pelvic abscess.

1.45 A. True
B. True
C. True
D. True
E. True

Staphylococcus aureus is a common organism on the skin and commonly infects wounds. MRSA wound infection is usually caused by wound contamination through hospital staff who may be carriers of the organism. Anaerobic organisms exert their lethal effects by producing endo- and exotoxins. Infection with opportunistic organisms is a result of the patient's reduced immune defence. The development of incisional hernia is frequently caused by the release of proteolytic enzymes from the bacteria in the wound.

1.46 A. True
B. True
C. False
D. False
E. False

Keloid scars are more common in patients of Afro-Caribbean origin with dark complexions. Wound infections predispose to keloids. Steroid injection therapy into the scar may reduce the incidence of keloid formation. The type of wound closure, whether primary or secondary, does not usually increase or decrease keloid formation. Use of the local anaesthetic bupivacaine has no effect.

1.47 A. True
   B. False
   C. False
   D. True
   E. True
   F. False
   G. True

Tracheostomy is indicated in patients in need of long-term ventilation. It can be performed as a cutdown or percutaneous mini-tracheostomy, which does not need to be done in the operating theatre. It does not require formal surgical closure when it is no longer needed. The recommended position of incision is at the level of the second and third rings of the trachea. Tracheostomy can be used to help in weaning patients off a ventilator and does not prevent speech in patients with the use of a speechbox. Scrupulous postoperative care is essential to avoid mechanical and infective complications.

1.48 A. False
   B. True
   C. True
   D. False
   E. False

A change in plasma viscosity is not diagnostic of DVT. A Doppler ultrasound scan and venography can be used in DVT diagnosis. It can also be diagnosed by radioactive ^{125}I-fibrinogen uptake. Homans' sign, where there is pain in the calf when the foot is forcefully dorsiflexed, is usually positive and a venous thermogram is usually negative.

1.49 A. False
   B. True
   C. True
   D. True
   E. False

Slow-release morphine patches and diamorphine are used for inpatients and are not suitable for day surgery patients. Diclofenac is a non-steroidal antiinflammatory drug and very useful for day surgery patients' analgesia. Local injection of the anaesthetic bupivacaine with adrenaline reduces postoperative pain. Metronidazole therapy reduces infection rates and thus reduces the pain caused by wound infection.

1.50 A. False
   B. False
   C. True
   D. True
   E. True

The Argon laser is used for photocoagulation of diabetic retinopathy. A CO_2 laser is used for the avascular excision of tumours. The Nd-YAG laser is used to arrest gastrointestinal bleeding and for palliative debulking of oesophageal tumours. A dye (tunable) photodynamic laser is used for the destruction of tumours after administration of a photosensitizing agent which is selectively taken up by tumour cells.

1.51 Theme: Lung masses
   1. E
   2. B
   3. C

1.52 **1.** F
 2. A
 3. D

High temperature steam is suitable for porous packed instruments which withstand heat. Dry heat is less efficient but may be used for solid objects, non-aqueous liquids and airtight containers. Ethylene oxide is used where heat sterilization is not possible, for example with delicate electrical and endoscopic equipment. Irradiation with gamma rays or accelerated electrons is useful for the sterilization of large batches of single-use items such as syringes or giving sets. Low temperature steam (without formaldehyde) and boiling water may be used for disinfection but not for sterilization.

1.53 **1.** C
 2. B
 3. E

The American Society of Anesthesiologists (ASA) status was originally introduced to predict the likely outcome of patients admitted to the intensive care unit. It is now widely used for the preoperative assessment of patients.

ASA 1 – Healthy patient.
ASA 2 – Mild systemic disease: no functional limitation.
ASA 3 – Severe systemic disease: definite functional limitation.
ASA 4 – Severe systemic disease that is a constant threat to life.
ASA 5 – Moribund patient not expected to survive 24 h with or without surgery.

Perioperative management (II)

2.1 **A.** True
     B. True
     C. False
     D. False
     E. False

Diabetes mellitus is a potent risk factor for cardiovascular and cerebrovascular disease. Insulin dependent diabetics should be assessed preoperatively for autonomic neuropathy (lying and standing BP) as this leads to lability of blood pressure during surgery. Perioperatively, lactate-containing solution (such as Hartmann's) should be avoided. Hourly perioperative monitoring of blood glucose is required because urinary glucose changes are too delayed.

2.2 **A.** False
     B. False
     C. True
     D. True
     E. False

A routine preoperative chest X-ray is required for all patients over the age of 65, and smokers over the age of 50. Patients with active lung disease or malignant disease processes also require X-ray. Patients having cardiac or thoracic surgery should also have a preoperative X-ray.

2.3 **A.** False
  B. True
  C. True
  D. True
  E. False

MRI should not be performed if the patient has metal implants including pacemakers and surgical clips (most clips now used are titanium). Previous eye injuries in patients working with power tools require orbital X-ray to exclude metallic foreign bodies. Iodinated contrast media used in CT scanning are replaced by paramagnetic agents (gadolinium) in MRI.

2.4 **A.** False
  B. True
  C. False
  D. False
  E. True

Patients of Afro-Caribbean or Indian extraction are at risk of sickle-cell disease. Northern Europeans, Australians and Scandinavians are at minimal risk.

2.5 **A.** True
  B. False
  C. True
  D. False
  E. False

ECG recordings are needed for patients over the age of 60 and those with documented or suspected cardiac disease. Hypertensive patients or those receiving treatment with cardiac drugs also need preoperative recordings. Surgery associated with cardiac complications such as abdominal aneurysm or thoracic surgery also require ECG.

2.6 **A.** False
  B. True
  C. True
  D. True
  E. True

Fresh frozen plasma is prepared from pooled donation, and although screened in the UK as such it may still transmit Hepatitis B and C. It contains most clotting factors but is depleted of fibrinogen and Factor VIII. Its use is recommended for the replacement of clotting factors, reversal of warfarinization and the treatment of DIC.

2.7 **A.** True
  B. False
  C. False
  D. False
  E. False

Antibiotic prophylaxis in colorectal surgery is effective in reducing superficial wound infection. Regimens should be active against Gram-negative and Gram-positive bacteria and should be administered to ensure maximum tissue concentration at the time of surgery. There is no evidence to suggest that the new second-generation cephalosporins are more efficacious than first generation. A single dose or short regimens (<24 h) are as efficacious as long-term use and may be associated with fewer side effects.

Universal acceptance of a regimen should be prevented to minimize the development of antiobiotic resistant bacteria. Research suggests guidelines should be developed locally.

2.8 **A.** True
    B. False
    C. False
    D. False
    E. False

Superficial abscesses commence when an innoculum of bacteria is surrounded by an accumulation of neutrophils, to constitute a fluctuant mass with a pyogenic membrane. Most are the result of infection with *Staphylococcus aureus*.

Prompt drainage of an abscess reduces the surrounding pressure effect and allows for evacuation of pus and the bacterial load. Antibiotic treatment is not generally required unless there is evidence of systemic toxicity. Perianal abscess should not be treated conservatively. Breast abscesses may be treated by repeated needle aspiration and antibiotics, but may require draining, preferably through a circumareolar or circumferential incision.

2.9 **A.** False
    B. False
    C. True
    D. False
    E. True

Universal precautions recommended by the Occupational Safety and Health Organization include the use of double gloves, impermeable gowns and waterproof footwear. Sharps should be passed to the scrub nurse/operating surgeon in a kidney dish and disposed of in appropriate sharps bins which are destroyed by incineration. Needles should not be resheathed; all needle-stick injuries should be reported to Occupational Health.

2.10 A. False
  B. True
  C. True
  D. False
  E. False

Monopolar surgical diathermy involves the passage of high frequency alternating current (400 kHz–1 MHz) through the body tissue. When the current is locally concentrated (forceps tip) temperatures of up to 1000°C are generated. Current returns to earth via the patient electrode which should measure at least 70 cm² to cause minimal local heating.

Monopolar diathermy may affect pacemakers, causing arrhythmia or arrest. Current may pass down pacemaker wires to cause myocardial burns. However, diathermy may be used if the electrode is placed such that current used does not pass near the pacemaker. A cardiology opinion should be sought. Bipolar diathermy cannot be used for cutting.

2.11 A. False
  B. False
  C. True
  D. False
  E. False

Lasers are devices for producing highly directional beams of coherent, monochromatic, in phase, electromagnetic radiation. Energy is pumped into the lasing medium (which is commonly gaseous, but may be crystalline Nd-YAG) to excite the atoms. As a result of an electron spontaneously falling from the excited to the ground state, a photon is emitted. The lasing medium determines the wavelength of the emitted light.

The Nd-YAG laser penetrates 3–5 mm. It is useful for coagulating large tissue volumes and leaves behind an eschar of damaged tissue.

2.12 A. False
   B. True
   C. True
   D. False
   E. True

Thrombocytopaenia may result from a reduction in the production of platelets from the megakaryocytes in the bone marrow or increased consumption of platelets in the circulation or hypersplenism.

Hypoplasia or infiltration of the bone marrow leads to failure of maturation of the platelets. Disseminated intravascular coagulation, idiopathic thrombocytopaenia and certain viral infections lead to an increased consumption of platelets. Sequestration of platelets within the spleen occurs in lymphoma and liver disease.

2.13 A. True
   B. False
   C. True
   D. False
   E. True

Risks to hypertensive patients undergoing surgery may arise because of sudden and uncontrolled changes in the blood pressure. Excessive blood loss or hypotension as a result of visceral stimulation may lead to perioperative myocardial infarction, or cerebrovascular accident. Poor perfusion of kidneys may lead to renal damage.

2.14 A. True
   B. False
   C. False
   D. True
   E. False

Morbidly obese patients are defined as being over twice the ideal weight for their height. Surgical disease may be difficult to diagnose in the obese patient. These patients are immobile both pre- and postoperatively and are prone to deep venous thrombosis. They tend to suffer from hypertension, diabetes and arthritis, which may be exacerbated by postoperative immobility. They are prone to chest infections and hypercarbia and may require prolonged postoperative ventilation. Laparoscopic surgery is not contraindicated, and may be easier for both patient and surgeon.

2.15 A. False
   B. True
   C. True
   D. False
   E. False

Perioperative complications of patients with obstructive jaundice may be prevented by the use of crystalloids to maintain adequate fluid balance, urine output and prevent acute tubular necrosis. 500 ml of 20% mannitol may be used perioperatively. Sepsis is reduced by the administration of intravenous antiobiotics. Haematoma formation and haemorrhage are reduced by the correction of the prothrombin time with intramuscular or intravenous Vitamin K. Early relief of jaundice by biliary stenting reduces later surgical morbidity.

2.16 A. False
 B. True
 C. True
 D. False
 E. False

Infection rates are reduced by appropriate scrubbing, gowning and gloving techniques. However, a 3–5 min scrub is only required at the start of a list; a shorter 1–2 min scrub is sufficient between cases.

In the operating theatre, the number of colony-forming units per m^3 theatre air increases the more personnel there are in the theatre. Gentle tissue-handling techniques to avoid bruising and haematoma formation do reduce infection rates. Braided ligatures trap organisms in their interstices.

There is no evidence that the use of theatre masks alters the rate of wound infection. It is advisable for staff with upper respiratory tract infections to wear a mask.

2.17 A. False
 B. False
 C. False
 D. True
 E. True

Minor surgical incisons are usually made parallel to the skin tension lines to reduce scarring. Contracted scars are usually lengthened using the technique of Z-plasty; advancement flaps made by undermining adjacent skin are most commonly used for closing defects left after lesion excision.

Several nerves are prone to injury at the time of minor surgery. The spinal accessory nerve is in the posterior triangle of the neck.

Infected wounds may be left open to heal by secondary intention, closed later by delayed primary suture or closed loosely with interrupted sutures.

Keloid scarring is differentiated from hypertrophic scarring by the fact that it extends beyond the original scar.

2.18 A. True
    B. True
    C. False
    D. True
    E. False

Keloid scars occur after minor surgery as a result of excess collagen accumulating in the wound. In hypertrophic scars this stays within the margins of the original scar; keloid scarring extends beyond these limits. A tendency to form keloids is genetically predetermined. They are commoner in pigmented skin. They often overlie the sternum and deltoid regions.

2.19 A. False
    B. False
    C. False
    D. False
    E. False

A clean contaminated operation is when the incision is made through non-infected skin under controlled conditions. It includes the opening of any hollow viscus (with the exception of the bowel) with minimal contamination which is controlled. Clean contaminated operations are associated with <8% of infection. A single shot or three doses of antibiotic prophylaxis is sufficient.

2.20 A. True
    B. True
    C. True
    D. True
    E. True

There are many contributing risk factors. Patient factors include: immunosuppression (infective or therapeutic), diabetes, intercurrent illness, obesity, nutritional status and trauma. Emergency operations lead to higher rates of postoperative infection than do elective ones. Poor tissue handling on the part of the surgeon leads to tissue ischaemia and bruising. Overtight sutures predispose to ischaemia. A prolonged preoperative stay in hospital leads to alterations in the body flora predisposing to more virulent organisms.

2.21 A. True
B. True
C. True
D. True
E. True

The treatment of choice for *S. aureus* is flucloxacillin. Clindamycin, cefuroxime and some of the other cephalosporins have antistaphylococcal activity as well as the glycopeptides (vancomycin and teicoplanin). *Staphylococcus aureus* that is not sensitive to methicillin is termed MRSA – methicillin resistant.

2.22 A. False
B. False
C. False
D. False
E. False

Endogenous infections are caused by infection with organisms carried by the patient, mainly Gram-positive Staphylococci and diptheroids. Antibiotic treatment may alter the normal flora leading to replacement by organisms likely to be conditional pathogens in the surgical context. Organisms acquired from theatre air (and therefore reduced by laminar flow) or hospital personnel are exogenous infections.

2.23 A. True
B. False
C. True
D. True
E. True

Causes of immunocompromise may be congenital – agammaglobulinaemia or hypogammaglobulinaemia – or acquired. Patients are immunocompromised after surgery or major trauma; when infected with HIV; when suffering from blood dyscrasias, myelofibrosis or leukaemia; or post splenectomy. Immunosuppressive drugs include azathioprine and cyclosporin A; steroids also suppress immunity. Severe medical conditions – renal failure, jaundice, diabetes and advanced malignancy – reduce the immune response.

2.24 A. False
   B. False
   C. True
   D. False
   E. False

Round-bodied needles are used for suturing bowel. Triangular or 'cutting' needles are used for suturing skin. Blunt needles are now available for the mass closure of wounds, reducing the likelihood of injury to the surgeon's fingers during closure. There is no evidence to support the use of non-absorbable sutures for mass closure. J needles are useful in tight corners, for instance the closure of a laparoscopy wound or femoral hernia repair, but are not usually employed for subcuticular suturing.

2.25 A. True
   B. True
   C. False
   D. True
   E. True

Increasing abdominal distension and pain are early signs of possible anastomotic leakage. Elevation of the white count with associated pyrexia is suspicious. Ten days postoperatively, any free gas introduced at the time of surgery will have been absorbed by the peritoneal cavity.

Discharge of pus through the vagina, particularly in patients who have previously undergone hysterectomy, is indicative of the presence of a pelvic haematoma which has become infected. Such collections frequently discharge through the anastomosis resulting in a leak.

2.26 A. False
   B. False
   C. False
   D. True
   E. True

T-tube drains are commonly used to drain the bile duct after exploration for stones but may also be used for the oesophagus after perforation or the ureter. They are made of latex rubber. This is resistant to the hardening effects of bile and encourages a fibrous reaction around the drainage tract. The tube is left in for at least ten days to develop a fibrous tract to the skin; if any bile leaks after removal this drains along the tract to the skin and reduces the likelihood of peritonitis. Because T-tubes are very soft they are easily occluded as they pass through the abdominal wall and when they are secured in place.

2.27 A. True
   B. False
   C. False
   D. False
   E. False

A posterolateral thoracotomy through the 5th intercostal space is at the level of the lung hilum and gives good access to the lung hilum and the mid-portion of the oesophagus.
   The great vessels are better accessed through a median sternotomy. The incision which is limited posteriorly by the vertebral bodies should be along the upper border of the rib to avoid damage to the intercostal neurovascular bundle. The thoracotomy is closed using No. 1 nylon pericostal sutures.

2.28 A. True
    B. True
    C. True
    D. True
    E. True

Lignocaine is a commonly used local anaesthetic agent. It is alkaline in solution and has a local vasodilatory effect which is often counteracted by the use of adrenaline.

Lignocaine blocks the uptake of sodium into nerves. The maximum safe dose for a 70 kg man is 150 g – a 1% solution contains 100 mg per 10 ml (1 g per 100 ml). Lignocaine toxicity should be suspected if the patient complains of tingling around the mouth, followed by drowsiness and slurred speech which leads to convulsions and then coma.

2.29 A. False
    B. False
    C. False
    D. False
    E. True

Local anaesthetic injections are painful, but a number of manoeuvres are useful in reducing the pain felt at the time of injection. Warn the patient before you inject the anaesthetic and use the thinnest needle possible. Neutralizing the alkaline pH (not acid pH) helps, as does warming the anaesthetic. The concurrent administration of adrenaline worsens the vasoconstrictive effect.

2.30 1. E
    2. F

The first history is consistent with a diagnosis of gallstones. Abdominal ultrasound is the investigation most likely to confirm this suspicion. Gallstones are not always seen on CT scans.

The second history, in a postoperative patient who has been poorly mobile, is likely be secondary to a pulmonary embolism. While signs of right heart strain may be identified on an ECG they are not always present. Arterial hypoxia with hypocapnia secondary to hyperventilation is a more useful indicator of recent pulmonary embolism.

2.31 **1.** B
2. D
3. H

2.32 **1.** C
2. J
3. E

Streptococci are Gram-positive cocci which cause cellulitis and necrotizing fasciitis. *Strep. pneuomiae* is the commonest form of community acquired respiratory infection. *Strep. milleri* is an important cause of abscess in the liver and brain.

2.33 **1.** B
2. F
3. D

Fine needle aspiration is the first-line biopsy technique when the tissue architecture is not required to make a diagnosis, for example a breast lump. Core needle biopsies give more architectural information but risk the development of a haematoma or damage to underlying structures. Endoscopic biopsy is a useful technique for lesions within a hollow viscus such as the colon or stomach; however these tissue samples are often small and superficial.

Hollow tubes that are difficult to access endoscopically and shed cells easily such as the pancreas and bile duct may be biopsied using brush cytology.

Incision biopsy is employed when the lesion is fixed and not easily removed without damage to surrounding structures. Excision biopsies are those where the lesion is removed in its entirety, preventing cell spillage in the case of melanoma, and allowing study of the capsule of lymph nodes and thyroid nodules for example.

Answers

Trauma

3.1 **A.** False
  B. True
  C. False
  D. False
  E. False

The initial assessment of the multiply injured patient should follow the ATLS-type primary survey format. Airway with cervical spine control is the first priority, with ventilation control and chest injury management coming second, and shock assessment and management third. Pulse oximetry is an invaluable tool for monitoring oxygenation during initial resuscitation. Pulse oximetry may read falsely low in the patient who is cold or shocked.

Cervical spine control is always indicated in the multiply injured. External haemorrhage control forms part of the primary survey and is a component of shock management. Ischaemic limbs are not immediately life threatening and should not distract from resuscitating vital functions.

3.2 **A.** False
  B. False
  C. False
  D. False
  E. False

All multiply injured patients should initially receive high concentrations of oxygen; those who do not have chest injuries, shock or coma can have their oxygen therapy altered later. Airway obstruction following trauma is usually associated with coma: that is, the tongue obstructs the oropharynx because of loss of muscular tone in the unconscious patient. The oropharyngeal airway is tolerated well in the comatose patient, but is extremely irritant to the semicomatose or conscious patient. The nasopharyngeal airway is better tolerated in the semiconscious patient. The laryngeal mask airway does not protect the tracheobronchial tree from aspiration of stomach contents. The endotracheal tube can be passed effectively in either spontaneously breathing patients or apnoeic patients.

3.3 **A.** True
  B. False
  C. False
  D. True
  E. False

The acute loss of 750 ml of blood from an adult patient results in tachycardia and vasoconstriction. Blood pressure is maintained until over 1500 ml have been lost. The vasoconstriction naturally causes skin pallor with reduced capillary refill. Oliguria is not seen until over 1500 ml blood loss has occurred. During the initial stages of shock the haematocrit will remain unaltered as whole blood is lost. Only after infusion of crystalloid or colloid will the haematocrit drop.

3.4 **A.** True
  B. True
  C. False
  D. False
  E. True

The patient with tension pneumothorax is usually tachypnoeic and agitated, tachycardic as a result of pain, anxious, hypoxic, hypercarbic and has decreased venous return. There is splinting of movement of the affected hemithorax, which may appear hyperinflated, with decreased breath sounds and an increased and tympanitic percussion note. Neck veins are distended secondary to mediastinal compression (there may be decreased cardiac output because of reduction in venous return), and the trachea is deviated.

3.5 **A.** True
  B. True
  C. False
  D. False
  E. True

Tension pneumothorax rapidly results in respiratory failure, and the mediastinal collapse and distortion results in shock. The healthy lung is compressed and diaphragmatic excursion is inhibited resulting in hypoxia and hypercarbia.

Open pneumothorax produces immediate equilibration between intrathoracic pressure and atmospheric pressure. When the defect is the same dimension as the tracheal diameter, then air will preferentially pass through the defect rather than through the trachea itself.

Flail chest implies multiple rib fractures with loss of rib cage integrity, resulting in abnormal chest wall movements. There is ineffective ventilation on the injured side, as each respiratory effort results in flail segment movement rather than 'fresh air' movement. There is marked pulmonary contusion underlying the flail segment, which is perfused but not ventilated, and the V/Q mismatch causes profound desaturation.

Isolated pulmonary contusion usually takes 6–12 h to develop, whereupon respiratory compromise will become manifest. Diaphragmatic rupture similarly results in gradual herniation of abdominal contents and it can take days before there is life-threatening respiratory embarrassment.

3.6 **A.** False
B. True
C. True
D. True
E. True

3.7 **A.** True
B. True
C. True
D. False
E. False

In tension pneumothorax, there exists a one-way air leak from lung parenchyma to pleural space, and more tension develops with each breath. IPPV will worsen such patients. In patients with open pneumothorax, IPPV allows effective ventilation of both lungs, with the lung on the injured side gradually reinflating after occlusion of the chest wall defect.

Pulmonary contusion patients may derive some benefit from maximizing oxygenation of the partially consolidated lung. Carbon dioxide control can be achieved by hyperventilation of healthy lung to compensate for carbon dioxide retention caused by injured lung.

In flail chest, IPPV will result in efficient ventilation of both lungs.

There is considerable risk of converting a small simple pneumothorax into a large tension pneumothorax, by the application of IPPV. These patients usually require chest drainage. A large diaphragmatic rupture allows herniation of abdominal contents into the chest cavity causing interference with lung expansion. These are reversed by IPPV.

With mediastinal traversing wounds there is often both haemo- and pneumothorax. Chest drainage will be useful.

Surgical emphysema often develops in the absence of clinical pneumothorax, and its resolution is unaffected by chest drainage. If mechanical ventilation is required, however, then the emphysematous side should be drained in order to prevent conversion of a subclinical simple pneumothorax into a life-threatening tension pneumothorax.

3.8 **A.** True
    B. False
    C. False
    D. False
    E. False

Resuscitative thoracotomy (immediate thoracotomy) is performed through a left anterior thoracotomy at the 5th intercostal space. It is only indicated in patients with penetrating thoracic injuries who are pulseless but with myocardial electrical activity (electromechanical dissociation). Those with a precordial stab wound who demonstrate signs of cardiac tamponade, that is, low cardiac output and distended neck veins, will respond to infused volume and should undergo exploration in theatre unless moribund.

Patients with blunt chest trauma who present in electromechanical dissociation are unlikely to benefit from such surgery unless there is clear evidence of cardiac tamponade.

In patients with massive haemothorax, the need for surgery is determined by ongoing blood losses rather than the initial drainage.

3.9 **A.** True
    B. True
    C. False
    D. False
    E. True

3.10 A. True
  B. False
  C. False
  D. True
  E. True

Diagnostic peritoneal lavage (DPL) is indicated in unstable patients with multiple sites of injury or in the unstable comatose patient, but should not be performed in the patient with obvious need for laparotomy. In general peritoneal lavage is used in unstable (shocked) patients, and other forms of imaging, usually CT, are used for stable patients. CT can detect solid organ damage or intraperitoneal blood, but will miss many visceral and diaphragmatic injuries.

   DPL is highly sensitive for intra-abdominal bleeding but less useful at detecting visceral, diaphragmatic or retroperitoneal injury. The bladder should be emptied and the stomach aspirated before commencing. After insertion of the PD catheter, free aspiration of blood or gastrointestinal contents is clearly positive and mandates a laparotomy. Lavage fluid (approximately 10 ml/kg) is introduced. A red cell count of greater than 100 000 cells/mm³ or a white cell count of greater than 500 cells/mm³ is deemed to be positive.

3.11 A. False
  B. False
  C. False
  D. True
  E. False

Gunshot wounds to the abdomen invariably result in extensive serious intra-abdominal injury. Such patients always require laparotomy. Bullet wounds tend to injure the organs with greatest presenting surface area, such as bowel, stomach and liver, so the injury patterns differ from those commonly associated with blunt injury. As visceral injuries are so common, it is recognized that CT or DPL are often falsely negative with such injuries, hence the requirement for exploration in all cases. Finally these patients often sustain major haemorrhagic injuries and cannot be stabilized without surgery (which is a part of resuscitation), so it is often inappropriate to carry out the usual X-ray series associated with blunt trauma management.

3.12 A. False
 B. True
 C. True
 D. True
 E. True

Pelvic fractures are notoriously difficult to detect by clinical examination alone, apart from the 'open book' type of grossly displaced fracture.

Peritoneal lavage is useful in determining if the patient has also sustained intra-abdominal injury and clinical signs of tenderness are often obscured by the adjacent skeletal fractures. DPL can, however, be falsely positive because of communication with the pelvic and retroperitoneal haematoma, and it should be carried out above the umbilicus to avoid the preperitoneal haematoma which often arises from the pelvic fracture.

The management for the massive haemorrhage associated with open pelvic fractures is external skeletal fixation and closure of the pelvis to tamponade the bleeding points. Severe pelvic crush fractures are often compound to rectal or less commonly vaginal or bladder mucosa. Such rectal injuries invariably require a defunctioning colostomy as part of their management, and there is considerable risk of pelvic sepsis in such patients.

3.13 A. True
   B. True
   C. False
   D. False
   E. True

Intracranial pressure (ICP) is normally around 10 mmHg, and pressure above 20 mmHg is considered abnormal. Smaller intracranial space occupying lesions can be accommodated without a rise in ICP by compensatory reduction in venous intracranial volume and CSF intracranial volume. As the space-occupying lesion enlarges, a point of decompensation is reached whereupon the ICP will rapidly rise to dangerous levels.

Cerebral perfusion pressure is calculated by subtracting the ICP from the mean arterial blood pressure (MAP). Clearly patients who have raised ICP, or reduced MAP, or both, will have diminished cerebral perfusion pressure.

Cushing's reflex is seen in the patient with isolated raised ICP. Such patients develop hypertension in an attempt to maintain cerebral perfusion pressure, and there is a secondary bradycardia mediated via a baroreceptor reflex.

Autoregulation describes the mechanism whereby the patient with an uninjured brain can maintain an even cerebral blood flow despite wide variation in arterial blood pressure. The patient with an isolated head injury is sometimes hypertensive because of Cushing's reflex, but is rarely hypotensive as a direct result of the head injury itself. In such hypotensive comatose patients always search for occult blood loss to explain the hypotension, and other causes of hypotension should also be considered.

3.14 A. True
  B. False
  C. False
  D. False
  E. False

Pyramidal (voluntary) motor function is controlled by the precentral gyrus, that is, the gyrus just anterior to the central sulcus and forming part of the frontal lobe. The oculomotor nerve (III) supplies all the orbital muscles except superior oblique (trochlear nerve: IV) and lateral rectus (abducent nerve: VI). The nerve carries parasympathetic fibres which causes pupillary and ciliary constriction. Compression of the oculomotor nerve causes pupillary dilatation.

CSF is manufactured by the choroid plexus within the lateral ventricles, then circulates via the third ventricle and fourth ventricle to the subarachnoid space. The fluid is returned to the bloodstream principally through the arachnoid villi of the superior sagittal sinus. The posterior cranial fossa describes the inferoposterior aspect of the cranial cavity, and this contains the cerebellum, pons and medulla. It is roofed in by the tentorium cerebelli on which lie the occipital lobes of the cerebral hemispheres.

3.15 A. True
  B. True
  C. True
  D. True
  E. True

3.16 A. False
B. True
C. True
D. True
E. True

Extradural haematoma may occur after a relatively minor primary brain injury. The lesion most commonly occurs when a meningeal artery tears because of a skull fracture, but it can also result from venous sinus injury. The presence of skull fracture therefore greatly increases the risk of extradural haematoma. Basal skull fractures are also associated with an increased risk of haematoma.

An open skull fracture implies a dural tear associated with a basal or vault fracture, communicating with a scalp wound or air sinus. Patients with CSF rhinorrhoea have an open fracture and are at significant risk of meningeal infection. They require antibiotic prophylaxis, principally against pneumococcus.

The patient may suffer transitory loss of consciousness. The lucid interval describes the period following recovery from the primary brain concussion and preceding the coma caused by the secondary brain injury (compression). Clinical signs include ipsilateral pupillary dilatation and contralateral motor weakness.

Patients require rapid control of intracranial hypertension by intubation and modest hyperventilation, with mannitol infusion. Computed tomography will show a biconvex radio-opaque lesion, as the spread of the extradural haematoma is limited by the adherence of the dura to the overlying cranium.

Subdural haematoma tends to be associated with significant cerebral injury and is often caused by the tearing of a bridging vein between the cerebral cortex and venous sinus. The prognosis for these injuries is usually much worse than that associated with extradural haematoma.

3.17 A. True
   B. False
   C. False
   D. False
   E. False

Most patients with a GCS of less than 13 require intubation
and CT scanning. Intubation is carried out in order to:
1. Provide a robust airway.
2. Protect the tracheobronchial tree from aspiration.
3. Provide enhanced oxygenation.
4. Control carbon dioxide levels by hyperventilation.
If the patient with head injury is hypotensive, do not attribute
their hypotension to their injury – they usually have an
extracranial cause of hypotension.

   Following intubation, the patient will require
neuromuscular paralysis, to ease mechanical ventilation and
prevent surges in blood pressure which might otherwise occur
if the patient fights the ventilator. They will however continue
to demonstrate normal pupillary reflexes and these are the
only way of detecting a patient's deterioration pending
imaging by CT scan.

   Skull X-rays are not very helpful in the severely head
injured patient, especially where there is a clear indication for
CT scanning.

3.18 **A.** False
    B. True
    C. True
    D. False
    E. True

The spinal cord runs from the foramen magnum to the level of the second lumbar vertebrae whence it becomes the filum terminale, surrounded by the cauda equina. The subarachnoid space which contains CSF continues to sacral level.

The posterior column of the cord contains mainly ascending fibres associated with touch, pressure, vibration and proprioception from the same side of the body.

The spinothalamic tract is the principal afferent pathway transmitting sensation, and ascends in the lateral column of the cord (pain and temperature), and in the anterior column of the cord (touch), to reach the thalamus and thence the postcentral cortical gyrus. The fibres cross the cord prior to forming the columns.

The C6 dermatome includes the thumb and radial border of the hand and forearm, the C7 dermatome includes the middle finger, and the C8 dermatome includes the fifth finger and ulnar border of the hand and forearm.

The L3 myotome innervates knee extensors (and the knee jerk), the L4 myotome innervates ankle extension, the L5 myotome innervates hallux extension, and the S1 myotome innervates ankle flexion (and the ankle jerk).

3.19 A. False
   B. False
   C. True
   D. False
   E. False

Cervical spinal cord injury results in four main clinical effects:
1. Myotome-based weakness or paralysis below the level of the lesion.
2. Dermatome-based paraesthesia or anaesthesia below the level of the lesion.
3. Autonomic dysfunction caused by loss of sympathetic outflow.
4. Respiratory dysfunction caused by loss of intercostal function.
Patients remain flaccid and arreflexic for several weeks: this is known as spinal shock. After this period, spasticity and hyperreflexia supersede and are permanent. Sacral sparing of sensation tends to be associated with a slightly better prognosis.

   A cord lesion above T1 level effectively abolishes sympathetic outflow. Patients typically vasodilate and become hypotensive; the loss of cardiac accelerator fibres leaving unopposed vagal tone results in bradycardia. The hypotension is usually neurogenic rather than hypovolaemic in origin, although clearly blood loss can coexist with spinal injuries. The low cervical cord lesion denervates intercostal muscles, and ventilation is maintained by the phrenic nerve (C3, C4 and C5). These patients exhibit diaphragmatic breathing.

3.20 A. False
B. False
C. True
D. True
E. True

Most scoring systems are too cumbersome for field use or triage. The abbreviated injury scale (AIS) is an anatomical scoring system whereby individual injuries receive predetermined scores, ranging from 0 to 6 depending on severity.

The injury severity score (ISS) is an anatomical scoring system, related to AIS. Taking the three highest AIS scores in predetermined regions of the body, these are then squared and added together to produce the ISS. A score of 16 or over implies severe trauma.

The revised trauma score (RTS) is a physiological scoring system which analyses respiratory rate, systolic blood pressure and the Glasgow Coma Scale.

The combination of RTS and ISS, with other factors such as the age of patient, and whether the injury is blunt or penetrating, go to make up the TRISS methodology. TRISS effectively provides a statistical measure of probability of survival, applicable to the average patient with a particular injury pattern. It should not be used for individual survival predictions, however, but can be used to compare groups of patients with similar survival probabilities, in order to compare outcomes between differing centres, for example.

APACHE stands for Acute Physiology and Chronic Health Evaluation.

3.21 A. False
    B. False
    C. True
    D. False
    E. True

Split-skin grafting consists of epidermis and a variable thickness of dermis and contain adnexal remnants (hair follicles, sebaceous follicles and sweat gland remnants).

When a split-skin graft is transferred to its recipient site, it must reattach and revascularize, a process known as 'take'. This is usually evident in 3–4 days. Examples of good recipient sites include muscle, fascia and sometimes fat where the blood supply is good. Examples of poor recipient sites include bare cortical bone, bare cartilage and bare tendon, although the periosteum, perichondrium and paratenon will readily accept grafts.

Haematoma, shearing movements and bacteria such as *Streptococcus pyogenes* and *Pseudomonas aeruginosa* can result in graft failure.

Provided a skin graft is kept moist and at a low temperature (around 4° C) it can survive for up to three weeks.

3.22 **A.** True
      B. False
      C. True
      D. False
      E. False

A flap is transferred tissue which contains a vascular network of arteries, capillaries and veins, upon which flap survival depends. Skin itself only contains capillary buds and cannot therefore be transferred as a flap. Skin flaps do exist but also contain subcutaneous fascia, for example, fasciocutaneous, myocutaneous and osteomyocutaneous flaps.

Local flaps retain a vascular attachment during transfer, being rotated or advanced. A free flap can be moved to a remote site, with the artery and vein reanastomosed to vessels in the recipient area. Pedicled flaps are a variety of local flap where only the distal portion of the flap is transferred to the recipient site, leaving a bridge of tissue unattached to the recipient site, but which acts as a conduit for the blood supply to the distal portion. After a delay of around three weeks the distal portion of the flap will have established a local blood supply; the bridge of tissue can then be divided. In general all flaps leave a secondary defect after transfer, and this can either be primarily closed or skin grafted.

The Transverse Rectus Abdominis Myocutaneous (TRAM) flap can be used locally for breast reconstruction or transferred as a free flap for distal tibial coverage.

3.23 A. True
   B. True
   C. False
   D. False
   E. True
   F. False

Full thickness burns tend not to blister, presumably because blistering depends on an intact dermal blood supply exuding serum into the epidermal/dermal layer. Superficial partial thickness burns will heal in approximately ten days with minimal scarring. Burn area is usually calculated using Wallace's Rule of Nines formula. Fluid replacement is calculated by the Muir and Barclay formula, which includes surface area of burn wound as a percentage of total body surface area, and the weight of the patient. Upper airways can sustain direct thermal injury, lower airways (bronchi) can sustain chemically induced bronchospasm, and alveoli can sustain chemically induced pneumonitis.

Carboxyhaemoglobinaemia will not be detected by a pulse oximeter as it is misinterpreted as being oxyhaemoglobin. Most burn wounds are fairly sterile and do not require antibiotic prophylaxis.

3.24 A. False
    B. True
    C. False
    D. False
    E. False

The Le Fort I fracture is really a separation just above the maxillary teeth and therefore does not involve the orbits. The Le Fort II fracture extends from the pterygoid plate through the maxillary-zygomatic suture, then involving nasofrontal junction. The Le Fort III fracture describes a complete separation of all the facial bones, including the zygoma, from the base of the skull.

The higher fractures, Le Fort II and III, often involve the cribriform plate and result in CSF rhinorrhoea, and all three fractures tend to have some degree of epistaxis.

Oral intubation is the simplest and safest option. Nasal intubation may precipitate further haemorrhage and may cause contamination of the meninges where there has been a dural breach at the cribriform fascia.

Orthopantomogram is a panoramic tomogram of the mandible. Maxillary fractures are best demonstrated by occipitomental views and these are best taken with the patient standing.

3.25 A. True
     B. False
     C. False
     D. True
     E. False

Orbital blowout fractures occur through the thin orbital floor or medial orbital wall. There is often associated herniation of orbital contents into the fracture site – for example, orbital fat and ocular muscles.

In inferior orbital blowout, there is trapping of inferior rectus muscle, and elevation of the globe is limited, causing diplopia on upward gaze. There is usually no injury to the oculomotor nerve itself. There is often injury to the infraorbital nerve (a branch of the maxillary nerve, the second division of the trigeminal nerve) with resultant infraorbital paraesthesia. Occipitomental facial views often demonstrate a fluid level in the maxillary antrum with a 'hanging drop' sign in the antrum roof, where the orbital contents have herniated through the orbital floor. CT scans could completely miss the fracture and the herniated orbital contents.

3.26 A. False
     B. False
     C. False
     D. True
     E. True

When a missile passes through tissue it will cause direct damage to the tract of tissue through which it passes by laceration and crushing. This is known as the permanent cavity. As missiles are retarded by the body's tissues, there is energy transfer producing a temporary cavity. This forms a vacuum and sucks in air, debris and bacteria, collapsing a few milliseconds later. With very high velocity missiles there is extensive tissue damage as a result of temporary cavitation, and there is extensive bacterial contamination also. Temporary cavitation tends to cause devastating injury to more solid organs such as the liver, as their compliance is less.

Abdominal gunshot wounds invariably result in extensive tissue damage and laparotomy is mandatory. Cranial missile wounds quickly result in cerebral oedema, and ventilatory control is generally required.

3.27 A. True
B. False
C. False
D. False
E. False

The Primary Triage Officer is normally an ambulance officer who sorts casualties into priorities for treatment while at the scene.

All patients who can walk, or who clearly have simple lower limb injuries, are prioritized as requiring 'delayed' treatment and allowed to leave the scene. If a casualty does not breathe despite simple airway manoeuvres he is pronounced dead and not usually resuscitated: such casualties are known as 'expectant'. If breathing is present with airway support, or is present but is too fast or too slow (>30 or <10), or if the patient is clinically shocked, that is, pulse >120/min or capillary refill >2 s, then the casualty is prioritized for 'immediate' treatment. All remaining casualties who have a normal respiratory pattern, without airway support, and have normal circulation fall into the 'urgent' treatment category.

The Chief Triage Officer at the hospital is usually a senior emergency physician. The overall hospital response is co-ordinated by the Medical Co-ordinator. The Medical Incident Officer takes control at the incident scene.

3.28 A. False
B. False
C. False
D. False
E. False

Healing by second intention should not be used on facial wounds even where there is significant contamination, as it will produce a poor cosmetic result. Delayed presentation of wounds, even up to 24 h, makes little difference to the degree of contamination, and primary closure should be attempted. For most skin lacerations, however, antibiotic prophylaxis is unnecessary, especially with facial or hand wounds where blood supply is usually good. Glass foreign bodies are visible in well over 90% of cases, and soft tissue X-rays (reduced penetration) are often valuable in their detection. The commonest organism to infect skin wounds is *Staphylococcus aureus*.

3.29 A. False
   B. False
   C. True
   D. True
   E. True

The median nerve supplies the thenar muscles and the radial (lateral) two lumbricals. The ulnar nerve supplies the hypothenar muscles, the ulnar (medial) two lumbricals, and all the interossei and adductor pollicis. The radial nerve does not supply any of the intrinsic hand muscles.

The ulnar nerve supplies sensation to the one and a half ulnar digits, front and back; the median nerve supplies the three and a half radial digits on the flexor aspect; the radial nerve supplies the dorsal aspect of the radial aspect of the hand, especially the dorsum of the first web.

The radial nerve supplies all hand and digit extensors in the forearm. The musculocutaneous nerve supplies the elbow flexors including biceps and brachioradialis.

3.30 A. True
   B. False
   C. True
   D. True
   E. True

The femoral nerve supplies all knee extensors, pectineus and sartorius. Common peroneal nerve injury will produce foot drop, and sensory loss to the whole of the dorsum of the foot. The tibial nerve supplies the ankle flexors and the long digital flexors, all the short (intrinsic) foot muscles, and supplies sensation to the whole of the sole of the foot. The sciatic nerve is closely related to the posterior aspect of the hip joint where it is frequently injured.

3.31 A. True
   B. False
   C. False
   D. False
   E. True

An oblique or spiral fracture has a greater fracture surface area when compared to a transverse fracture, and clinical union will be reached more quickly. Comminuted fractures are however associated with more trauma to the surrounding soft tissues and this tends to result in delayed union. In general cancellous (spongy) bone, found at the metaphysis, heals faster than the dense cortical (compact) bone found at the diaphysis or midshaft region. While rigid internal fixation allows rapid mobilization, it does not in itself confer more rapid fracture healing, and actually inhibits callus formation with the result that true healing is slower. Epiphyseal injuries classically unite extremely rapidly as the epiphyseal growth plate lays down new metaphyseal bone rapidly.

3.32 A. True
   B. False
   C. False
   D. True
   E. True

Joint involvement sometimes leads to delayed union, possibly as a result of dilution of fracture haematoma by synovial fluid. Osteoporosis itself tends not to delay fracture healing, nor do many other bone pathologies such as Paget's disease. There is no significant difference in the rate of fracture healing between the young adult and the elderly.

Significant soft tissue injury is associated with delayed union, and this is most evident in compound fractures regardless of whether there is contamination or infection. In general excessive mobility delays healing. Conversely very rigid internal fixation can also remove the stimulus for healing. A small degree of movement is probably optimal, and many fixation devices are deliberately designed to allow micro-movement when the patient commences weightbearing, a process known as dynamization.

3.33 A. False
 B. False
 C. False
 D. False
 E. False

In femoral shaft fractures there is commonly adhesion between fracture site and overlying quadriceps muscle resulting in restriction of knee flexion caused by tethering of overlying muscle. The scaphoid receives its blood supply from the distal pole backwards, so a waist fracture often leads to avascular necrosis of the proximal pole. The talus also receives a distal blood supply, and the proximal talar body sometimes undergoes avascular necrosis following talar neck fractures. Fat embolism typically presents within a few days of injury. During the early stages of compartment syndrome the patient will have intense pain in the limb although swelling may not be obvious. They may not demonstrate the classical features of absent distal pulses or paraesthesia of the relevant peripheral nerve until much later.

3.34 1. E
 2. G

Patient X is maintaining a patent airway but nevertheless he may not possess protective airway reflexes to prevent tracheobronchial aspiration. He will clearly require ventilation to control his PCO_2 as neuroprotection. For these reasons, patients with a GCS of 12 or under usually require endotracheal intubation and mechanical ventilation. Nasotracheal intubation, in the presence of basal skull fracture or maxillary fracture, can cause meningeal contamination or even result in direct instrument trauma to the contents of the anterior cranial fossa, and should therefore be avoided.

   Patient Y will also require ventilation to manage his neurotrauma. If there is considerable difficult in placing an orotracheal tube, then cricothyroidotomy should be performed as an emergency room procedure.

3.35 **1.** E
     2. C
     3. D

Patient X has sustained only abdominal injury and exhibits evidence of hypovolaemic shock. This patient should proceed to immediate laparotomy without further tests or imaging. He is haemorrhaging briskly and control of major bleeds should be obtained as a priority. Diagnostic peritoneal lavage will only confirm that the patient is bleeding into the peritoneal cavity. Imaging in this patient will miss many important injuries and will also cause delay in haemorrhage control.

Patient Y has sustained an isolated injury but is quite stable. Imaging or DPL may allow a more elective approach to his management. CT scanning, ultrasound scanning or DPL will detect free intraperitoneal blood. All will however tend to miss bowel injury which often only becomes apparent after 12–24 h, when the patient becomes more tender and develops sepsis.

Patient Z is haemodynamically unstable, possibly as a result of the haemothorax and possibly as a result of her lower limb fractures. Her pelvis is intact. She may therefore have an intra-abdominal injury. There are no reliable local clinical signs as she is comatose. She will therefore require diagnostic peritoneal lavage.

3.36 **1.** B
     2. B

The younger man has sustained significant intrathoracic injury. He is showing signs of hypovolaemic shock and chest examination is suggestive of haemothorax. Such patients invariably require intercostal drainage, both to re-expand the lung by allowing drainage of haemo- and pneumothorax, and in order to monitor ongoing blood loss from the chest. There is little to be gained by waiting for a chest X-ray in such cases, which can be obtained following insertion of the intercostal tube.

The elderly man has a small simple pneumothorax. In the context of trauma, however, such a pneumothorax is at risk of enlarging or even becoming a tension pneumothorax. All traumatic pneumothoraces should therefore ideally be drained. In the elderly patient full lung expansion is also very important to prevent atelectasis and chest infection.

Intensive care

4.1 **A.** False
  B. False
  C. True
  D. True
  E. True

The right diaphragm normally lies at the level of the upper border of the 5th rib anteriorly and the left at the lower border of the 5th rib anteriorly. Indeed if the 7th ribs are cleared by the diaphragm anteriorly, then the lung fields are pathologically hyperinflated. The carina lies at a level between the 4th and 5th thoracic vertebrae behind the sternal angle. The hila of the lung can be pulled up or down by fibrosis or collapse of the lung. The oblique fissure can be traced on a lateral X-ray from the body of the 4th thoracic vertebra to the anterior margin of the diaphragm. If a line is drawn from the mid-point of the left atrial appendage to the right cardiophrenic angle, then the aortic valve will lie above the line and the mitral valve will lie below it.

4.2 **A.** True
B. False
C. True
D. False
E. False

The lung volumes often seem to cause confusion. They are best understood with reference to the diagram below:

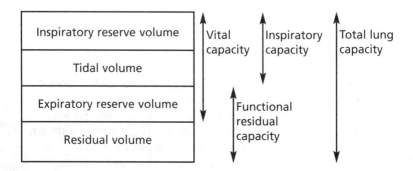

Of all the volumes and capacities FRC is the most important when concerned with anaesthesia and surgery. FRC is linearly related to height. For the same body height, males have an FRC about 10% higher than females. Age has no effect on FRC; it falls by about 25% when moving from the erect to the supine position.

Lung disease can have a profound effect on FRC. It is reduced by increased elastic recoil of the lungs and chest wall, for example in fibrotic lung disease, bony deformities and obesity. FRC will rise with diseases that produce reduced elastic recoil of the lung, emphysema and asthma being the best examples.

Although not strictly a lung capacity, the closing capacity is very important in understanding why the arterial PO_2 falls with age. The closing capacity is the lung volume at which airway closure begins. If this occurs during normal tidal breathing, then some of the blood perfusing the lungs will not come into contact with ventilated tissue. This represents a shunt and may result in arterial hypoxaemia.

4.3 **A.** False
    B. True
    C. True
    D. True
    E. False

The normal recording rate of an ECG is 25 mm/s. The PR interval is prolonged in first degree heart block and shortened in WPW syndrome.

The normal QRS complex is 0.06–0.10 s. Between 0.10 and 0.12 s there is an incomplete bundle branch block (BBB) which is of little clinical significance. QRS complex above 0.12 s indicates a BBB, hyperkalaemia or ventricular ectopic foci.

The normal cardiac axis is –30° to +90°. More negative than this indicates left axis deviation and more positive, right axis deviation.

4.4 **A.** True
    B. True
    C. False
    D. False
    E. True

The proximal port opens in the right atrium, which is used as a CVP monitor and is also used to inject the solution for cardiac output studies.

The distal port opens in the pulmonary artery, and is used to measure pulmonary artery pressures, pulmonary artery wedge pressures and also to sample mixed venous blood.

The balloon inflation port opens to a lumen that terminates within the balloon. Finally, the thermister port incorporates a temperature-sensitive wire that terminates approximately 4–6 cm proximal to the tip of the catheter.

From samples of mixed venous blood taken from the catheter, estimations of oxygen delivery and consumption can be made.

In patients with pulmonary disease resulting in pulmonary hypertension, the pulmonary artery wedge pressure will not give an accurate representation of left atrial pressures, as a result of high pulmonary vascular resistance. In these situations the pulmonary artery diastolic pressure gives a better indication of left atrial filling pressures.

4.5 **A.** False
    B. False
    C. True
    D. False
    E. True

This is not a massive blood transfusion, since only around 14% of this patient's circulating blood volume has been replaced. Massive transfusion is defined as the replacement of a patient's entire circulating blood volume in a short period of time.

Complications of any transfusion include:

1. A haemolytic reaction caused by ABO incompatibility. In its severest form the reaction is immediate and is associated with intravascular haemolysis, as a result of complement activating antibodies of the IgM or IgG class. Its treatment is to stop the transfusion and give supportive therapy.
2. Allergic reactions to white cells and plasma proteins
3. Infections (such as HbsAg, CMV, EB virus, HIV, malaria, syphilis and bacterial infections) are now less common than they were because of screening, but can still occur.
4. Air embolus can occur when giving any intravenous infusion – 0.5 ml/kg is enough to cause death.
5. Thrombophlebitis can occur with any transfusion.
6. Microaggregate embolism can also occur with any transfusion but may be prevented with the use of filters.

4.6 **A.** True
B. False
C. False
D. True
E. False

The question is asking what conditions cause shunting or areas of low V/Q. Shunting is defined as that part of the lung which is not ventilated but is perfused. The V/Q in this situation is zero. Areas of the lung with low ventilation which are perfused will result in areas of low V/Q. In both these cases, the net result is that mixed venous blood fails to exchange with gas in the lungs and thus returns to the left side of the circulation virtually unchanged. Here it combines with arterial blood that has been oxygenated during its passage through the lung. Because of the shape of the oxyhaemoglobin dissociation curve, and because mixed venous blood only has an oxygen content of 5 ml/dl blood compared to 20 ml/dl of blood, shunting causes a significant desaturation of arterial blood.

The alveolar partial pressure of oxygen (P_AO_2) is inversely proportional to alveolar ventilation and is not related to shunting. (P_aO_2 is the partial pressure of oxygen in the arterial blood.) Any condition that causes a reduction in alveolar ventilation will cause the P_AO_2 to fall but the P_aO_2 also falls, but by the same degree such that the $P_AO_2:P_aO_2$ gradient remains the same.

In a shunt situation, the P_AO_2 remains the same but the P_aO_2 falls such that the $P_AO_2:P_aO_2$ gradient rises.

4.7 **A.** False
B. True
C. True
D. False
E. True

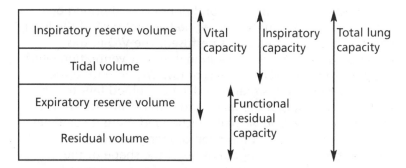

Compare with question 4.2. Spirometry is unable to measure residual volume. Since functional residual capacity and total lung capacity include residual volume in their measurement, spirometry is also unable to measure these parameters. All other volumes and capacities of the lung can be estimated using the spirometer.

In addition, the spirometer can estimate forced expired volume in 1 s (FEV_1). The ratio of FEV_1 to vital capacity should exceed 75% in normal subjects. If it is below this it may indicate airways obstruction due to chronic obstructive airways disease or asthma. The ratio of FEV_1 to vital capacity is elevated (e.g. 90%) in restrictive lung disease, for example, as a result of fibrosing alveolitis or chest wall deformity.

4.8 **A.** True
  B. True
  C. True
  D. True
  E. False

A red light-emitting diode (660 nm) and an infrared light-emitting diode (940 nm) shine light through a finger (or ear) and a photocell detects the transmitted light. By measuring the ratio of absorption of the red to the infrared light, the saturation of haemoglobin can be estimated. A microprocessor is programmed to analyse the changes of light absorbence during the arterial pulsatile flow and ignore the non-pulsatile component of the signal caused by tissues and venous blood. In this manner, the pulse oximeter measures only the saturation of arterial blood.

The following may effect the accuracy of measurement of haemoglobin saturation (normally ± 2%): methaemoglobinaemia, carboxyhaemoglobin (hence inaccuracies in smokers), bilirubin, methylene blue, excessive vasoconstriction (hence inaccuracy in shock), excessive ambient light (it works well in darkened rooms), the shape of the oxyhaemoglobin dissociation curve (on the steep part of the curve at about 94% saturation readings become increasingly inaccurate) and movement artifact.

4.9 **A.** True
B. False
C. True
D. True
E. False

Three methods are available for measuring FRC.
1. In the nitrogen washout technique, the person being measured breathes 100% oxygen from FRC while nitrogen is collected in a container. From the concentration of nitrogen in the container and the volume of gas collected, the amount of nitrogen in litres can be estimated. Since the initial alveolar concentration of nitrogen is measured, the initial volume of the lung (that is, FRC) can be calculated. If, for example, 3.2 l of nitrogen was collected and the initial alveolar concentration of nitrogen was 80%, the FRC is 4 l.
2. In the helium dilution technique, the patient breathes into an apparatus into which a known concentration of helium is added. Since helium is not taken up by the body, the helium is effectively diluted by the patient's FRC. By measuring the new concentration of helium, the FRC can be estimated.
3. In body plethysmography, the patient is enclosed in an airtight box and attempts to breathe against an occluded airway. Pressure changes measured at the mouth correspond to alveolar pressure and the pressure change in the box is also measured. The plethysmograph is calibrated such that a given volume change is known to produce a given pressure change. By applying Boyle's Law lung volume can be calculated.

Fowler's method and the Bohr equation are used to derive physiological deadspace.

4.10 A. True
   B. False
   C. False
   D. True
   E. False

The patient receives a preset minute volume. In the intensive care unit, IPPV is usually known as continuous mandatory ventilation. If a patient is not paralysed then he may not synchronize with the ventilator in this setting, resulting in high airway pressures. In SIMV, the ventilator detects inspiratory effort by the patient, upon which a breath is initiated by the ventilator and thus there is improved synchronicity between the patient and the ventilator. In SIMV, even if the patient is paralysed, he will receive a preset minute volume (hence the term mandatory). In PSV, the ventilator also detects the patient's inspiratory effort and then assists the patient's breathing by giving additional positive pressure. In this case, the minute volume is not preset, so that in a paralysed patient, PSV will fail to ventilate the patient.

   Neither CPAP or PEEP are means of ventilating patients. CPAP is used in spontaneously breathing patients to keep the airways open at end-expiration (although the positive pressure is maintained throughout the ventilatory cycle). PEEP is used in ventilated patients to keep the airways open at end-expiration. The aim of both is to improve oxygenation by reducing shunt.

4.11 A. True
   B. True
   C. False
   D. False
   E. True

Cardiac output is increased as a result of an increased inotropic ($\pm$ chronotropic) effect. Vasodilation of the splanchnic vascular bed occurs and urine output is increased because of the increased cardiac output ($\pm$ increased renal blood flow). Dopamine can stimulate the chemoreceptor trigger zone (which lies outside the blood–brain barrier) causing nausea and vomiting.

4.12 A. False
  B. True
  C. False
  D. True
  E. True

Dextrose/saline (1 l) contains 31 mmol each of sodium and chloride ions and 40 g dextrose. It has a calculated osmolality of 286 mosmol/l (that is, nearly isotonic with plasma).

4.13 A. True
  B. True
  C. True
  D. True
  E. True

The daily water requirement may be calculated from the following equation:

$$1500 \text{ ml} + [(\text{weight (kg)} -20) \times 25] \text{ ml}$$

Sodium requirements are 1–2 mmol/kg/day, potassium requirements are 0.8–1 mmol/kg/day. Energy requirements are 30–40 kcal/kg/day and protein requirements are 1 g/kg/day. Fats should provide 30–50% of daily energy requirements. For a 70 kg patient 1 l of 0.9% sodium chloride and 1.5 l of 5% dextrose will provide the water and sodium. If 20 mmol potassium are added to the sodium chloride and 40 mmol potassium are added to the 5% dextrose then an adequate potassium intake will result. For patients starved for longer periods, nutrition must be achieved with either NG feeding or more rarely TPN.

4.14 A. True
  B. True
  C. False
  D. True
  E. False

A combination of clinical evaluation of the ECF, plasma osmolality and urine sodium concentration are used to establish the causes of hyponatraemia. Excessive hyerlipidaemia causes pseudohyponatraemia in a dilutional way, the total body sodium being normal and the patient euvolaemic. Hepatic cirrhosis is associated with oedema with water retention. Lithium antagonizes the effects of ADH on the renal tubules, causing a water diuresis in excess of the sodium excretion. Diarrhoea, in a patient who is not taking fluids (orally or intravenously), will result in hypernatraemia. However a patient with diarrhoea who is replacing the losses with salt-poor fluid will become hyponatraemic. In nephrogenic diabetes insipidus there is an impaired response to ADH on the renal tubules, causing a water diuresis in excess of the sodium excretion. In neurogenic diabetes insipidus there is impaired production of ADH from the posterior pituitary causing the same effect.

4.15 A. True
  B. True
  C. False
  D. True
  E. False

The Ramsay score grades a patient's level of sedation on a scale of 1–6, from highly agitated to deeply comatose. Midazolam has a short elimination half-life (approximately 90 min) which makes it a suitable agent for sedation on the ITU. Morphine is metabolized by the liver and excreted as glucuronides. It should therefore be used with caution in patients with impaired liver function. Unlike morphine, fentanyl is far more lipid soluble which accounts for its rapid uptake and distribution.

4.16 A. False
   B. True
   C. True
   D. True
   E. True

Salicylates stimulate the respiratory centre in the medulla resulting in increased respiratory rate and depth. A respiratory alkalosis might therefore be expected. The metabolic acidosis is thought to result from direct effects on intracellular metabolism with consequent increases in lactate and pyruvate levels. Hypokalaemia is also a presenting feature that may be worsened by bicarbonate therapy for the accompanying metabolic acidosis. Despite being an antipyretic in therapeutic dosage, one of the presenting signs of toxicity – especially in children – is fever.

4.17 A. False
   B. False
   C. True
   D. False
   E. True

CO poisoning is one of the more common types of poisoning, either deliberate or accidental. Because of its vastly greater binding capacity to the haemoglobin molecule (200 times greater) it results in impaired oxygen delivery to the tissues. The mainstay of therapy is oxygen with other appropriate supportive measures. Unfortunately COHb does not correlate well to severity; levels above 40%, however, indicate significant toxicity and usually present with CNS signs of confusion and drowsiness. The arterial oxygen concentration may be normal and does not reflect tissue hypoxia. Some reports recommend use of hyperbaric oxygen therapy in patients presenting with neurological signs. Severe CO poisoning may also have more longstanding implications such as persistent headache, personality change and other neuropsychiatric complaints.

4.18 **A.** True
  B. False
  C. False
  D. False
  E. True

A recent study showed statistically significant improvement in outcome in patients who received methylprednisolone (30 mg/kg bolus followed by infusion 5.4 mg/kg/h for 24 h) within 8 h of spinal injury. Because of unopposed parasympathetic activity bradycardia, vasodilatation and hypotension are the more usual cardiovascular problems seen in the acute stage. A much higher proportion (50%) have accompanying head injury. The benefit of hyperbaric oxygen therapy in decreasing tissue hypoxia has yet to be proven. Spinal injury patients are at increased risk of DVT so prophylactic measures should be commenced early.

4.19 **A.** False
  B. True
  C. False
  D. True
  E. False

Tetanus results from exposure to the exotoxin tetanospasmin produced by the Gram-positive *Clostridium tetani*. The micro-organism gains access via surgical or traumatic wounds, however in many cases the portal of entry may not be obvious. The toxin then proceeds to interfere with neural transmission of spinal inhibitory neurons. Ninety per cent of cases present within 15 days of infection. Human immunoglobulin only helps to neutralize circulating toxin so that the cornerstone of treatment is wound debridement where appropriate and general supportive measures such as analgesia, sedation and cardiovascular and respiratory support if required. Laryngospasm may necessitate intubation and ventilation. Patients may also require treatment for surges in sympathetic discharge that can cause hypertension and tachycardia. Patients are not immune post recovery and therefore should receive immunization therapy before discharge.

4.20 A. False
  B. False
  C. True
  D. True
  E. False

Like most diuretics, dopamine inhibits Na/K ATPase, thereby decreasing sodium reabsorption producing a natriuresis. Dobutamine has no effect at renal dopaminergic receptors. An increase in urine output with this inotrope is secondary to improved cardiac output. Loop diuretics act on the thick ascending loop of Henle also by inhibiting Na/K ATPase cotransport mechanism.

4.21 A. False
  B. True
  C. True
  D. True
  E. True

Vancomycin is a bactericidal agent active only against Gram-positive bacteria, particularly aerobes. It has no clinical activity against Gram-negative bacteria. It is active against MRSA and all forms of coagulase negative *Staph.* (CNS). Nephrotoxicity is very uncommon but doses should be reduced in patients with renal impairment. If vancomycin is infused too quickly it may produce extensive flushing of face and neck – the so-called Red Man syndrome. While the oral preparation is effective against *Clost. difficile*, most workers would recommend the use of metronidazole as first-line treatment unless very severe.

4.22 A. False
  B. False
  C. True
  D. True
  E. True

Alcohol and epilepsy are prominent features in cases of near drowning. The immediate problems arise from asphyxia. Even small amounts of aspirated water (2.5 ml/kg) can have a dramatic effect on lung function progressing to ARDS. Steroids and prophylactic antibiotics are of unproven benefit. Theoretically serum electrolytes fall with fresh water near drowning and rise with saltwater, but are often not significantly disturbed.

4.23 A. True
   B. False
   C. True
   D. True
   E. True

The ECG changes are more likely with an acute rise in potassium rather than with chronic elevation. Elevated serum potassium causes a widening of the QRS interval. Urgent treatment is indicated if ECG changes occur in the presence of hyperkalaemia. The initial short-term measures include insulin glucose, bicarbonate and calcium chloride followed by cation exchange resins to remove the potassium from the body.

4.24 A. True
   B. True
   C. False
   D. True
   E. True

Cerebral blood flow as measured by the Fick principle approximates at 50 ml/100 g/min, roughly 12% of the cardiac output. Autoregulation allows for the maintenance of a constant blood flow despite alterations in arterial blood pressure. It is probably related to a myogenic response. Normotensive autoregulation occurs between 60–130 mean arterial pressure (MAP). Hyperkalaemia results in dilatation of the cerebral vessels. Cerebral blood flow increases linearly with increasing carbon dioxide tension. Conversely alterations in cerebral blood flow related to oxygen tension only occur at P_aO_2 <7.5 kPa. Transcranial Doppler, PET scanning and Xe 113 are methods used in clinical practice to determine cerebral blood flow.

4.25 A. False
　　　B. True
　　　C. True
　　　D. False
　　　E. True

The IABP is a form of circulatory assistance for the failing heart. It improves cardiac performance by decreasing afterload, reducing systemic vascular resistance and by augmenting aortic diastolic pressure. It may be used in those patients with failing left ventricle from MI, post bypass or mechanical defects. Inflation of the balloon may be timed either with the patient's ECG (the R wave) or arterial blood pressure trace. Severe aortic regurgitation, aneurysm and severe peripheral vascular disease are relative contraindications to its use.

4.26 A. True
　　　B. True
　　　C. True
　　　D. False
　　　E. False

Acidosis reduces renal potassium excretion. In acidosis, the plasma bicarbonate concentration is low and therefore chloride ions are preferentially reabsorbed from the kidney. Acute metabolic acidosis will cause a compensatory hyperventilation and the P_aCO_2 falls. Tetany is seen in alkalosis when there is reduced serum-free ionized calcium. Acidosis is associated with hyperphosphataemia.

4.27 A. False
　　　B. False
　　　C. True
　　　D. False
　　　E. True

In the UK, a flat EEG is not a requirement for the diagnosis of brain death. There must be absent motor responses when testing the cranial nerve distribution, although spinal reflexes may still be present. If brainstem death has occurred then the oculocephalic reflex is absent and therefore when the head is moved from side to side, the eyes remain fixed. The doctor making the diagnosis must have been fully registered for five years.

4.28 A. True
  B. True
  C. False
  D. True
  E. True

Rhabdomyolysis is a clinical syndrome resulting from severe skeletal muscle injury. There may be a multitude of aetiologies but alcohol, compression injuries and seizures appear most common. Alcohol itself has a direct myotoxic effect. Metabolic acidosis, hyperkalaemia, hyperuricaemia and hyperphosphataemia may occur. Hypocalcaemia is common in the acute phase of the injury (60%). Large-volume fluid resuscitation is needed to prevent renal failure and to treat the biochemical abnormalities. CPK, which is produced in skeletal muscle, is released into the blood and causes levels to rise when damage occurs.

4.29 A. False
  B. True
  C. False
  D. True
  E. True

The acute phase of ARDS is characterized by exudative lung lesions from diffuse pulmonary capillary leak as opposed to lung oedema from hydrostatic pressure increases as seen in cardiac failure and fluid overload. Pulmonary compliance and the surfactant function are decreased. Oxygen free radical scavengers may be of benefit but this is still largely unproven. ARDS is associated with conditions such as pancreatitis, sepsis and trauma.

4.30 A. True
  B. True
  C. True
  D. True
  E. False

Prolonged intestinal obstruction leads to dehydration and uraemia. The patient usually develops a metabolic acidosis and a compensatory respiratory alkalosis. The patient might well be hypoxic if only breathing room air, but there is no particular reason for hyperglycaemia.

4.31 A. True
  B. False
  C. True
  D. True
  E. True

In haemorrhage the central venous pressure (CVP) is low, as is the blood pressure, since there is a reduced intravascular volume. In all the other situations listed above there is either pump failure (myocardial infarction, congestive cardiac failure), or obstruction to the pulmonary circulation (pulmonary embolism, tension pneumothorax). In these instances therefore the damming back of blood in the venous circulation leads to an elevated CVP, while there is hypotension caused by the pump failure or the obstruction to blood flow.

4.32 A. False
  B. True
  C. True
  D. False
  E. True

Transurethral resection (TUR) syndrome may occur as a result of absorption of the irrigating fluid used. The volume absorbed is reduced if the height of the irrigating fluid is <60 cm and if the duration of surgery is <60 min. About 20 ml/h is normally absorbed. The fluid used is iso-osmotic 1.5% glycine solution. As it is iso-osmotic its absorption does not cause haemolysis. Glycine is used as it has good optical properties without conducting electricity, thereby reducing the risk of burns.

Glycine is an inhibitory neurotransmitter and thus its absorption causes CNS effects such as confusion, seizures, cerebral oedema and irritability. Absorption of large volumes of irrigating fluid into the vascular space leads to signs of pulmonary oedema and heart failure, often with hypotension and, paradoxically, bradycardia.

Classically there is hyponatraemia because of dilution. Management involves administering oxygen and possibly a diuretic, together with fluid restriction. The serum sodium must be corrected slowly as too rapid correction may lead to central pontine myelinolysis, which has a very high mortality. Disseminated intravascular coagulation can occur as part of the TUR syndrome.

4.33 A. True
   B. True
   C. False
   D. True
   E. True

Fat embolism occurs with fracture or operation on a long bone. A triad of respiratory compromise, cerebral dysfunction and petechial haemorrhages may be seen. There may be a pyrexia and ARDS or DIC can supervene in severe cases. It is associated with a mortality of 10–20%.

4.34 A. True
   B. True
   C. False
   D. True
   E. False

Cushing syndrome leads to hypokalaemia and a metabolic alkalosis. A gastrocolic fistula leads to loss of gastric acid, as does pyloric stenosis. Acetazolamide is a carbonic anhydrase inhibitor which may be used to treat metabolic alkalosis. Hyperkalaemia is associated with metabolic acidosis.

4.35 A. True
   B. True
   C. True
   D. True
   E. True

All of the above are potential complications of the siting of an arterial line. Thrombus may form at the site and may then embolize to the lungs or the brain if there is a patent foramen ovale, which is present in about 10% of the population.

4.36 A. True
    B. True
    C. True
    D. True
    E. False

The combination of hypotension and bradycardia suggests neurogenic shock and is caused by the loss of sympathetic vasomotor tone and the cardioaccelerator fibres. Although ultimately there will be signs of spasticity, because of upper motor neuron damage, initially there is spinal shock. This is manifest as arreflexic flaccidity of the limbs. Damage to the phrenic nerve (C3, C4, C5) occurs with high cervical cord injuries and leads to paralysis of the diaphragm. Lower lesions may only affect the intercostal muscles with less respiratory impairment.

4.37 A. True
    B. True
    C. True
    D. True
    E. False

DIC is a consumptive coagulopathy that may be triggered by many disorders. The result is consumption of platelets, fibrinogen and clotting factors with, paradoxically, widespread deposition of thrombus in the microvasculature of vital organs such as the kidney and brain. This thrombus activates thrombolysis and perpetuates the coagulopathy. The management, in essence, entails replacing what is missing – that is, platelets, fibrinogen (cryoprecipitate) and clotting factors (FFP).

It may occur with haemolytic transfusion reactions, following prostatectomy and in any septic patient.

4.38 A. False
    B. True
    C. True
    D. True
    E. True

Acute liver failure may be caused by viral hepatitis (Hepatitis A, B, C, CMV or EBV), alcohol, paracetamol or other toxins and, rarely, halothane. The commonest cause in the UK is paracetamol overdose. Indicators of a poor prognosis include a prothrombin time >3 × control, bilirubin >300 μmol/l and a pH <7.3.

    The liver enzymes alanine and aspartate aminotransferase (ALT and AST) are characteristically elevated and are sensitive markers of hepatocellular damage.

4.39 A. True
    B. True
    C. False
    D. False
    E. False

The oxyhaemoglobin dissociation curve is shifted to the right by decreased pH, raised PCO_2, raised temperature, raised levels of 2,3 DPG (as in chronic anaemia), altitude and hypoxia.

    The oxyhaemoglobin dissociation curve is shifted to the left by decreased pH, low PCO_2, hypothermia, and reduced levels of 2,3 DPG. The curve also shifts to the left in carbon monoxide poisoning and in the presence of HbF or other high affinity haemoglobins.

4.40 A. True
    B. True
    C. False
    D. False
    E. True

Vomiting leads to loss of HCl from the stomach, leading to a metabolic alkalosis. The resulting dehydration causes a raised blood urea. The kidney attempts to compensate by conserving hydrogen ions in exchange for potassium, hence the alkaline urine and the low plasma potassium.

4.41 A. True
B. False
C. False
D. False
E. True

At rest, the interior of the cell is negatively charged with respect to the exterior. This is because of an unequal ion distribution across the cell membrane, with potassium being mainly an intracellular ion and sodium being predominantly extracellular. The PR interval is prolonged in first degree heart block and the QT interval is prolonged in hypocalcaemia.

4.42 A. False
B. True
C. ~~True~~ F.
D. True
E. True

Problems in the postoperative period following a thyroidectomy may be immediate or occur once the patient is back on the ward. Among the immediate complications is wound haematoma. The surgeon will usually close the thyroidectomy scar with either clips or staples, and the patient is nursed with a set of instruments at the bedside should it be necessary to quickly evacuate a haematoma which might otherwise lead to tracheal compression and respiratory embarrassment. Another immediate complication that can occur is tracheal collapse.

Hypocalcaemia, resulting from removal of one or more of the parathyroid glands at surgery, tends to occur in the early postoperative period, but not immediately.

Thyroid crisis can occur intraoperatively or at any time in the postoperative period. Untreated, it may result in coma and be fatal. It usually presents with tachycardia, pyrexia, confusion and abdominal pain and requires treatment with beta-blockers and antithyroid drugs.

Laryngeal stridor may occur as a result of oedema or direct damage to one or both of the recurrent laryngeal nerves.

4.43 **A.** True
    B. False
    C. False
    D. False
    E. False

In effective mouth to mouth resuscitation the percentage of inspired oxygen is about 14%. The patient's expired CO_2 will be much greater than 2% because he is likely to have been apnoeic for some time.

    The patient will have both a respiratory and metabolic acidosis, the result of apnoea and anaerobic tissue metabolism, respectively. The pH of the blood will be less than 7.4, which is the normal plasma pH.

    The mixed venous oxygen saturation (SvO_2) in a normal individual is about 75%. In a patient receiving effective mouth to mouth resuscitation the SvO_2 would be unlikely to be greater than 75%.

4.44 **A.** False
    B. True
    C. True
    D. True
    E. True

Mannitol is a sugar, not an alcohol. It may be used to prevent hepatorenal syndrome in jaundiced patients, and in patients with cerebral oedema. Because it is a hypertonic solution it draws cerebral oedema into the vascular compartment by osmosis. This may, however, lead to circulatory overload. Also, if the blood–brain barrier is damaged and permeable there may be a paradoxical worsening of neurological status after administration of mannitol.

4.45 A. True
   B. True
   C. True
   D. True
   E. False

Bronchospasm may be pharmacologically precipitated. Morphine can cause histamine release which may then cause bronchospasm and wheeze. Pethidine has a lesser (but still possible) potential for histamine release, and may be preferred to morphine as an analgesic in an asthmatic patient. Stimulation of the trachea or carina by an endotracheal tube may lead to bronchospasm. 'Cardiac asthma' produces wheeze and can be confused with bronchospasm. Volatile agents cause bronchodilation and can be used in cases of severe, refractory bronchospasm.

4.46 A. False
   B. False
   C. True
   D. True
   E. True

All sedatives reduce BMR. It is increased by 14% for every °C rise in temperature. Basal metabolic rate is measured with the subject at rest and is therefore unaffected by exercise. BMR falls with age; it is increased by pain and anxiety.

4.47 A. False
   B. True
   C. False
   D. True

Naloxone is an antagonist at all opioid receptors and will therefore reverse pethidine. Naloxone causes no rise in blood pressure in normal individuals. The mechanism of naloxone inducing pulmonary oedema is not known.

4.48 1. D
2. B

The 46-year-old ex-smoker has acute metabolic alkalosis. The blood gas features of this condition are a high pH (> 7.44), normal PCO_2 and a high SBE (normal SBE = ± 2 meq/l). Chronic bronchitis is associated with a high PCO_2, a high SBE and normal/low pH. Pain and anxiety cause hyperventilation causing acute respiratory alkalosis, with reduction in the PCO_2, rise in pH and normal SBE. If the conditions become chronic, the kidneys respond by excreting bicarbonate and the SBE falls, with a subsequent fall in the pH. If prolonged, obstructive nephropathy (for example, a blocked catheter) could cause early post-renal failure with a metabolic acidosis. Renal tubular acidosis produces a metabolic acidosis. Aspirin overdose causes a combined metabolic acidosis and respiratory alkalosis. Hypokalaemia is the commonest cause of acute metabolic alkalosis. At the renal tubular level, the low K ion concentration causes H ions to be exchanged for Na with a resultant net loss of H ions and a metabolic alkalosis. This is exacerbated at the general cellular level where H ions are pumped into cells (in place of K ions) in exchange for sodium ions. This patient was probably on an intravenous infusion containing no potassium. It should be noted that the plasma potassium may be in the low/normal region. In cases like this, the SBE gives a better indication of potassium than the serum potassium.

The younger patient has an acute respiratory alkalosis. Probably the commonest cause of this condition in hospital is pain, causing stimulation of the respiratory system. None of the other conditions could produce blood gases like this.

4.49   **1.**   D
        2.   F
        3.   A

In the first patient, tension pneumothorax would be associated with desaturation of haemoglobin and an elevated CVP. Severe dehydration would tend to cause a more gradual onset of hypotension and the CVP would be low. Sepsis could easily produce a clinical picture like this. Acute onset of atrial fibrillation could produce hypotension due to the acute loss of the atrial component (30%) of ventricular filling but is not likely in a 28-year-old, as is an MI. PE would be associated with a drop in saturation and a rise in CVP.

With the thoracotomy patient, tension pneumothorax would be associated with desaturation of haemoglobin and an elevated CVP. Severe dehydration would tend to cause a more gradual onset of hypotension and the CVP would be low. Acute onset of atrial fibrillation could produce hypotension caused by the acute loss of the atrial component (30%) of ventricular filling and is the most likely diagnosis in a post-thoracotomy patient. Absence of ST changes on the ECG makes a diagnosis of MI unlikely. PE would be associated with a drop in saturation and a rise in CVP.

With the female patient, a pneumothorax is unlikely (but not impossible) using an internal jugular approach. It would also be associated with reduced air entry on the affected side. Sepsis and dehydration are not associated with a high CVP. The most likely diagnosis is a pulmonary embolus, unrelated to the CVP line insertion.

4.50 1. C
     2. B

In oliguric patients, such as in question 1, (= urine output < 0.5 ml/kg/h) assume dehydration unless proved otherwise. The immediate management is to administer 250–500 ml boluses of crystalloid or colloid and monitor changes in urine output. Better still, place a central line and go on the CVP. Accepted practice is to measure the CVP and then improve it by 3 cm H_2O with 250 ml fluid boluses and then watch the urine output. If it does not improve then increase the CVP by a further 3 cm H_2O and so on. The actual number is not as important as changes in a given value. In cases of dehydration, this technique should restore the urine output to normal if there is no renal damage. In cases of sepsis, it may take very large amounts of fluid to cause a change in CVP and this may not improve the urine output. The treatment usually requires inotropes.

Patient 2 has probably suffered blunt chest trauma and his cardiac function is compromised. He is adequately filled so the treatment of choice is dobutamine to increase inotropism and chronotropism. Although not in the list of options, a transoesophageal echo or pulmonary artery catheter could be useful in his management.

4.51 **1.** C
2. E
3. D

Adrenaline has approximately equal potency at alpha- and beta-adrenoceptors and causes an increase in cardiac output. Ephedrine is an indirectly acting sympathomimetic, causing release of adrenaline and noradrenaline from nerve endings with a smaller direct effect and increasing cardiac output. Noradrenaline has its major effect at alpha-adrenoceptors and causes peripheral vasoconstriction with a reflex bradycardia, thus decreasing cardiac output. GTN reduces the preload in cardiac failure and improves cardiac function in these patients. Dobutamine is active against beta- and alpha-adrenoceptors. Its main effect is on the heart where it causes an increase in cardiac output and it can be associated with a reduction in total peripheral resistance.

Patient 1 is septic and her SVR is very low. She requires noradrenaline to vasoconstrict her in order to increase her blood pressure.

Patient 2 has cardiac failure. He has a low cardiac output and a high SVR. The treatment of choice from the list is dobutamine. GTN may be useful but may compromise his (already low) blood pressure and would probably be started after the dobutamine.

The third patient also has cardiac failure but because her blood pressure is normal, she would benefit from GTN.

Neoplasia, the breast and techniques and outcome of surgery

NEOPLASIA

5.1 **A.** True
B. False
C. False
D. True
E. False

Lung cancer is the primary cause of cancer deaths in men and women. Despite a fall in incidence in men (but not women) there has been an increase in deaths over the last 60 years. Stomach and uterine cancer mortality has dropped, pancreatic has risen. Although the incidence of breast cancer has risen, improvements in treatment have kept the number of deaths basically steady.

5.2 **A.** True
B. False
C. True
D. False
E. False
F. True
G. False
H. False

Gastric cancer is associated with males, with low socio-economic groups, with Japanese ethnicity, a diet high in salt and nitrates and low in fruit and vegetables, and belonging to blood group A. There is evidence of a strong familial tendency though no specific gene has yet been isolated.

5.3 **A.** True
B. False
C. True
D. False
E. True
F. False

There are associations with diets high in red meats, saturated fatty acids and low in fibre. Fifty per cent of tumours arise in the rectum, and 25% in the sigmoid colon. HNPCC tumours are usually right sided and often mucinous.

5.4 **A.** False
B. False
C. True
D. True
E. True

Malignant melanoma is associated with solar damage caused by ultraviolet radiation. It is commonly seen on the legs of women and the trunks of men. It is seen more commonly in albinos, fair-skinned and red-haired people. Incidence increases with proximity to the Equator. There is an association with dysplastic naevus syndrome.

5.5 **A.** False
  B. False
  C. True
  D. True
  E. True
  F. False

Peutz–Jeghers is a rare inherited autosomal dominant condition where multiple hamartomatous polyps are found in the small intestine. Patients often have characteristic circumoral pigmentation. The polyps may ulcerate, bleed, cause anaemia and intussception. Malignant change is rarely seen but the condition is not *per se* premalignant.

5.6 **A.** False
  B. False
  C. True
  D. True
  E. True

Benign tumours have an expansile growth pattern while malignant tumours have an infiltrative growth pattern. Malignant tumours have an increase in the nuclear/cytoplasmic ratio and show nuclear pleomorphism (variation in size, shape and staining). Both benign and malignant tumours have an increased mitotic rate.

5.7 **A.** False
  B. False
  C. True
  D. True
  E. True

Adenomas arise from ductal or glandular epithelium as opposed to papillomas which can arise from squamous, transitional or columnar epithelium. They are usually rounded, can be polypoid, have a capsule and compress normal tissues around them.

5.8 **A.** False
  B. True
  C. False
  D. True
  E. True

K-ras is a GTP binding cytoplasmic signal transducer and is mutated in 60–70% of colorectal cancers. Tumours need a blood supply for their continued growth. Angiogenesis is stimulated by fibroblast-like growth factor, angiogenin, TNF alpha and TGF alpha. It is inhibited by TNF beta and angiostatin.

The process of metastasis requires the tumour cells to decrease their own adhesion, bind receptors in lymphatic or venous basement membranes and extracellular matrix and then by use of proteases such as metalloproteinases to dissolve the basement membrane. Normal cell adhesion is maintained by desmosomes, the negative charge on the cell surface and cadherins. Loss of cadherins in a cell line promotes invasion.

5.9 **A.** False
  B. False
  C. True
  D. False
  E. True

5.10 **A.** False
  B. True
  C. True
  D. True
  E. True

Lung cancer is the primary cause of death from malignancy in men and women, although its incidence is decreasing in men and increasing in women. It is associated with cigarette smoking, asbestos, uranium, arsenic and haematite exposure. Screening programmes with radiographs and sputum cytology have been shown to be ineffective. Ten per cent are incidental findings on chest X-ray. Paraneoplastic ectopic ADH secretion can produce hyponatraemia.

5.11 **A.** False
    B. True
    C. True
    D. False
    E. True

Oat cell tumours are highly malignant, often disseminated at diagnosis and have a 10% survival at two years. They are rarely amenable to surgery in comparison with the l0–15% of non-small cell tumours. There is some if not complete response to chemotherapeutic agents but not radiotherapy. Ectopic ACTH secretion produces a raised serum cortisol and Cushing syndrome.

Neurological symptoms are produced by brain secondaries and Pancoast's tumour in the lung apex producing brachial plexopathy and ptosis. Recurrent laryngeal nerve injury by direct tumour infiltration or lymph node pressure produces a hoarse voice. Paraneoplastic syndromes include inappropriate ADH secretion and ectopic ACTH production. Hypertrophic pulmonary osteoarthropathy produces painful wrists and clubbing.

5.12 **A.** False
    B. True
    C. False
    D. False
    E. True

In colorectal cancer 3% of patients will have a synchronous tumour at the time of diagnosis of the primary and 30% will have occult liver metastases. Right sided tumours often bleed as they are friable, causing an iron deficiency anaemia. They rarely obstruct because of the large bore of the caecum. Left sided tumours constrict in an annular fashion and obstruct earlier, also as a result of the more solid nature of the faeces in the left colon. They too can bleed, usually overtly, and produce mucus. Rectal tumours present with bright red bleeding, tenesmus, incontinence, rectal pain and urgency.

Faecal occult blood testing can be a useful screening tool although its specificity is low, with a high level of false positives as a result of diet. Regular sigmoidoscopy has shown poor potential as a population screening tool.

5.13 A. True
  B. True
  C. False
  D. True
  E. False

Renal cell cancer is more common in men, cigarette smokers and coffee drinkers. It is associated with cerebral and renal angiomas in the Von Hippel–Lindau syndrome. The tumours spread via the veins to the IVC and cannonball metastases to the lung are common.

5.14 A. True
  B. True
  C. False
  D. False
  E. False

Fever and a PUO are seen in 15%, anaemia in 30%, polycythaemia caused by erythropoietin production, a raised ESR in 50%, abnormal LFTs in 30%, myopathy, amyloid production, hypertension in 25% because of renin production or ischaemia, and hypercalcaemia as a result of ectopic parathormone production. A left sided varicocoele caused by the obstruction of the left testicular vein into the left renal vein (not IVC as on the right) is commonly described but rarely seen. Hypoglycaemia is seen with the rare juxtaglomerular haemangiopericytomas.

5.15 A. False
    B. True
    C. False
    D. True
    E. False

CA 153 is a sandwich two-monoclonal antibody marker of mucin. It is raised in 55–100% of advanced breast cancer, 10–46% of patients with primary disease and 10% of patients with early operable disease. However since it is raised in 2–30% of patients with benign breast disease it lacks the specificity and sensitivity for a screening tool. It is associated with a poorer prognosis if elevated preoperatively and is used in the early detection of relapse.

Neuron-specific enolas are raised in advanced small cell lung cancers and used in screening for neuroblastoma in children. Urinary 5H1AA is raised in patients with carcinoid tumours.

5.16 A. False
    B. False
    C. True
    D. True
    E. False

The retinoblastoma gene deletion is found on chromosome 13 and is inherited recessively. Oncogenes and their proteins are normal components of cellular molecular physiology and when over-expressed, mutated or modified function without regulation to up-regulate cell proliferation.

P53 is a tumour suppressor gene found on chromosome 17. It functions normally to recognize DNA damage and to stop the cell dividing until it repairs or allow cell death if the repair cannot be made. It is thus said to be the guardian of the genome. Mutations in p53 are common in tumours and the mutated form which has a long half-life binds to normal or wild-type p53 inactivating it and allowing uncontrolled cell proliferation. C-erb B2 is an abnormal growth factor receptor found in breast and gastric tumours which is like the epidermal growth factor receptor EGFR.

5.17 A. True
   B. False
   C. True
   D. True
   E. False
   F. True
   G. False

Breslow's thickness (rating melanomas of < 0.76 mm,
0.76–1.5 mm, >1.5 mm) has been shown to be a better
prognostic indicator than Clark's levels. Women are more
commonly affected. Ninety per cent arise in otherwise normal
skin and 10% in pre-existing naevi. A rapid increase in the size
of a mole, ulceration, bleeding, irregular outline, variation in
colour and itching arouse suspicion. Melanomas can also occur
in the eye, nasal cavities and gastrointestinal tract. The
superficial spreading type is most common (70%) and occurs
in covered and uncovered areas. The nodular type arises on
the trunk, lentigo maligna on the face of the elderly and the
acral lentiginous type on hairless skin in Asians and those with
a black skin. Lesions less than 0.76 mm should be excised with
a 1 cm margin, 0.76–1 mm with a 2 cm margin and >1 mm
with a 3 cm margin. Wider excision in deeper melanomas has
not been shown to be of added benefit. Women have a
better prognosis; this is probably related to tumour site and
stage at presentation. Melanomas on the hands, feet and
trunk have a worse prognosis than those elsewhere on the
limbs. Prognosis is worse if ulcerated, of high mitotic rate,
high histological grade or pedunculated.

5.18 A. True
  B. False
  C. False
  D. False
  E. False
  F. True
  G. True
  H. True

Hodgkin's disease has a bimodal age distribution; it peaks in the young (teens and mid-20s) and then increases again with age, especially in men. It is associated with higher social class, smoking in families and later birth position. Reed–Sternberg, bi- or multinucleate giant cells are classically seen but they can also be seen in infectious mononucleosis and drug reactions. Patients most commonly present with lymphadenopathy above the diaphragm (only 10% localized below). Generalized pruritis is seen as is pain in involved sites after alcohol ingestion. Systemic or 'B' symptoms such as weight loss, fever and night sweats are seen in 30% of cases. Five per cent of patients have localized extranodal disease at diagnosis. The ESR is increased in 30–50% and the bone marrow is involved in 5–15% of patients.

Enlarged mediastinal nodes are commonly involved in nodular sclerosing Hodgkin's and abdominal nodes are more commonly associated with mixed cellularity and lymphocyte depleted types.

The disease is staged by computerized tomography. Sixty per cent of those with disseminated disease can expect a cure from chemotherapy. Treated patients have a 15% risk of a second cancer 15 years after treatment, including non-Hodgkin's lymphoma, leukaemia, lung, stomach and melanoma.

5.19 A. True
B. True
C. False
D. True
E. False

In non-Hodgkin's lymphoma less than 10% are truly localized (stage 1) at presentation. Systemic chemotherapy is more commonly required than with Hodgkin's disease. Serum lactate dehydrogenase and age are prognostic factors as is tumour bulk. Forty per cent of patients have bone marrow involvement. Raised immunoglobulin levels in the lympho-plasmocytoid type produce increased plasma viscosity. Rapid tumour lysis in treatment can give uric acid nephropathy and renal failure. Primary gastrointestinal lymphoma is the most common extranodal presentation of the disease and the stomach is the most common site (55%).

5.20 A. True
B. False
C. True
D. False
E. True

Primary gastrointestinal lymphoma is rare but is the most common extranodal presentation of the disease. The stomach is involved in 55% of cases, the small bowel in 30% and it accounts for 0.1% of large bowel tumours. They are generally of high grade and require intensive combination chemotherapy postoperatively. Small bowel lymphoma is most common in the seventh decade of life and is sometimes multiple; they present with annular constrictions, and 30% present as perforation. Small bowel lymphoma is a recognized sequela of coeliac disease.

5.21 A. True
　　B. False
　　C. True
　　D. True
　　E. False
　　F. True
　　G. True

Early complications of radiotherapy include fatigue, anorexia, nausea and vomiting (especially with infradiaphragmatic radiation). Diarrhoea is seen as a result of radiation enteritis. Decreased saliva production produces an altered sense of taste. Skin reaction produces erythema and photosensitivity for six months. Thoracic treatment can produce dysphagia and cranial irradiation alopecia. Late complications include transient pneumonitis and respiratory disability.

Lhermitte syndrome produces numbness, paraesthesia and electric shock sensations in the lumbar region, upper and lower limbs, which lasts for up to six months.

Gonadal damage can produce azoospermia, permanent amenorrhea and premature menopause. Ischaemic heart disease can occur from coronary artery exposure and fibrosis and contracture of the bladder produces urinary problems.

5.22 A. False
  B. False
  C. True
  D. True
  E. True

Naturally occurring radioactive isotopes such as cobalt, caesium and iridium produce beta particles and electrons. They are often used for direct implantation into tissues – iridium wires for carcinoma of the tongue, vaginal caesium as cavity irradiation for carcinoma of the cervix and systemically as iodine 1-131 for carcinoma of the thyroid.

External beam radiotherapy uses a linear accelerator of electrons to produce high energy gamma rays which have greater tissue penetration than electrons. There is little scatter so the beam is sharp. The maximum dose is 1–2 cm below the skin therefore the skin gets a small dose.

High energy X-rays ionize body tissues, release electrons and produce DNA damage via an oxygen-dependent mechanism. Most of the DNA is repaired within hours.

Apoptosis or programmed cell death occurs in some normal cell lines (lymphoid and myeloid for example). The total dose is divided or fractionated and this allows normal tissue damage to repair and reoxygenation of hypoxic areas in tumours.

5.23 A. False
  B. True
  C. False
  D. False
  E. True

Seminomas and lymphomas are radiosensitive. Malignant melanomas, gliomas and sarcomas are radio-resistant. Adenocarcinomas and squamous cell tumours are relatively resistant but radiotherapy can have the advantage of preserving normal function where there are equivalent results with radiotherapy and surgery, for example carcinoma of the bladder and larynx. Some relatively radio-resistant tumours such as brainstem gliomas and sarcomas are irradiated because they are otherwise inoperable.

5.24 A. True
  B. False
  C. False
  D. True
  E. True

Adjuvant radiotherapy can be given pre- or postoperatively to improve local control (for example in breast or rectum). Preoperative radiotherapy may downstage extensive disease, reduce tumour seeding at the time of operation and can make accurate pathological staging difficult, but does not give an increase in surgical morbidity if surgery is performed within four weeks of treatment. Postoperatively it can be given prophylactically to high-risk areas such as the supraclavicular fossa in node-positive breast cancer. Palliative doses are often given as a single large fraction for recurrent chest wall metastases in breast cancer, bone pain, spinal cord compression, brain metastases in combination with dexamethasone and superior vena caval obstruction in lung cancer.

5.25 A. True
  B. False
  C. True
  D. False
  E. True

Chemotherapeutic agents aim to selectively destroy tumour cells while sparing normal tissues. Some drugs such as methotrexate and vinca alkaloids are cell phase dependent. Alkylating agents include cyclophosphamide, chlorambucil and cisplatinum; antimetabolites include methotrexate and 5-fluorouracil; and antitumour antibiotics include doxorubicin, mitozantrone, bleomycin and vincristine. Interleukin 2 has been used to treat metastatic renal cell cancer.

Combination regimens with different mechanisms of action and with minimal overlap in toxcitiy are used to reduce drug resistance and produce a synergistic effect. Vinca alkaloids (vincristine) and doxorubicin are said to be vesicant because if they extravasate from the vein, they produce massive tissue loss and damage owing to their toxicity.

5.26 A. True
  B. False
  C. False
  D. True
  E. True

Gastrointestinal toxicity – nausea and vomiting – are seen especially with cyclophosphamide and cisplatinum and act via the cortex, gut and chemoreceptor trigger zone. Alopecia is a particular problem with doxorubicin, cyclophosphamide and vincristine but practically never with 5-fluorouracil. Bleomycin is classically associated with pulmonary fibrosis, doxorubicin with cardiotoxicity and vincristine with peripheral neuropathy. Long-term treatment with melphalan and chlorambucil can lead to the development of acute leukaemia. Common side effects include bone marrow suppression, neutropenia, gonadal damage and sterility.

5.27 A. True
  B. False
  C. True
  D. True
  E. False

Chemotherapy has been shown to cure acute lymphoblastic leukaemia, choriocarcinoma, Ewing's sarcoma, Wilm's tumour and large-cell lymphoma. Local treatment followed by adjuvant chemotherapy can cure some breast tumours and osteogenic sarcoma. Ovarian and breast tumours and osteogenic sarcoma patients show prolonged survival following chemotherapy. Melanoma, soft-tissue sarcomas, colorectal tumours and tumours of the pancreas, kidney, thyroid and cervix are all poorly sensitive to chemotherapy.

5.28 A. False
B. False
C. False
D. True
E. False

In breast cancer if a tumour is oestrogen receptor positive, there is a 60% response to hormone manipulation; if both oestrogen and progesterone receptors are positive an 80% response. Tamoxifen is a partial agonist, partial antagonist of oestrogen and has been shown to prolong survival in breast cancer. In premenopausal women oophorectomy, LHRH antagonists and tamoxifen are used. In post-menopausal women aminoglutethimide and aromatase inhibitors are also used.

In carcinoma of the prostate, which is sensitive to testosterone and sex hormones, orchidectomy, LHRH antagonist and antiandrogens such as flutamide and cyproterone acetate are used. Gonadotrophin releasing hormone analogues such as goserelin are active but can give an initial disease flare.

5.29 A. False
   B. True
   C. False
   D. True
   E. False
   F. False

Tumour markers are not necessarily tumour specific but are secreted or shed in larger quantities by malignant cells. They are used for screening, diagnosis, as prognostic indicators and to monitor therapy.

CEA is raised in 5% of patients with Dukes' A carcinomas, 25% Dukes' B and 65% of Dukes' C tumours. A rising level predicts recurrence 11 months before it becomes clinically apparent.

CA l25 is a murine monoclonal antibody raised from carcinoma of the ovary. It is found in normal pleura, pericardium and peritoneum but not normal ovarian tissue. It is raised in 95% of patients with stage III or IV cancer of the ovary. It can also be raised in the first trimester of pregnancy, endometriosis and cirrhosis, and in 40% of advanced non-ovarian intra-abdominal cancers.

PSA is not specific and can be raised in benign prostatic hypertrophy.

Alpha fetoprotein is raised in 50–80% of patients with hepatocellular carcinoma and is used to screen high risk populations. CA l9-9 is raised in 75–90% of pancreatic carcinomas.

5.30 1. C
    2. E
    3. H
    4. A
    5. B

Urinary tract cancers are seen in aromatic dye workers, mesothelioma in asbestos workers, cancers of the nasal cavity in nickel miners, hepatocellular carcinoma in PVC workers and thyroid cancers are seen in association with exposure to ionizing radiation. There is a very high incidence of childhood thyroid cancer around the Chernobyl area.

5.31 1. B
2. D
3. A

Angiomyolipomas are tumours containing smooth muscle, blood vessels and fat. They are associated with tuberous sclerosis, are occasionally malignant and often bilateral. Juxtaglomerular tumours are small types of haemangiopericytomas that are small and situated in the renal cortex. They secrete renin, producing primary aldosteronism, with hypertension, hypernatraemia and hypokalaemia. They are associated with hypoglycaemia. Renal cell tumours present with loin pain, mass and haematuria, and often with fever, a raised ESR, anaemia or polycythaemia, myopathy and amyloid.

5.32 1. E
2. C
3. B

5.33 1. F
2. C
3. D

Although radiotherapy is very useful in the palliation of bone pain, with a young family and incipient pathological fracture anticipated from the >75% cortex erosion, prophylactic surgical fixation of the femur is indicated.

Liver capsule pain from stretching secondary to metastasis responds well to dexamethasone.

For pain from carcinoma of the pancreas failing to respond to opiates, a coeliac plexus block in the hands of a skilled person can give very good palliation.

THE BREAST

5.34 A. False
B. True
C. True
D. True
E. True

The breast is an ectodermal structure in embryological origin and is created through invagination of ectodermal cells into underlying mesenchyme. It arises from the 'milk lines' which run from axilla to groin, and along which accessory breasts may be seen in adulthood.

5.35 A. True
B. False
C. True
D. True
E. False

5.36 A. True
B. True
C. False
D. False
E. True

The long thoracic nerve (supplying the serratus anterior) and the thoracodorsal nerve (supplying the latissimus dorsi) should always be identified and avoided during surgery. Disruption to the former is associated with winging of the scapula, and the latter with weakness of shoulder adduction. The intercostobrachial nerve is sometimes sacrificed which can cause some numbness on the medial upper arm. The axillary vein marks the upper limit of dissection. Lymphoedema results from damage to lymphatics as a result of tumour, radiotherapy or surgery.

5.37 A. False
  B. False
  C. False
  D. False
  E. False

Mammography is most helpful in older and post-menopausal women in whom the glandular breast tissue is less dense. It requires compression of the breast against a plate. In younger women, ultrasound of the breasts may be more helpful.

5.38 A. False
  B. False
  C. True
  D. False
  E. True

Nipple discharge may be clear, milky, serous or bloodstained. Prolactinomas are anterior pituitary lesions which may present with nipple discharge. Intraductal papillomas are often associated with a bloody discharge. Fibrocystic disease can sometimes cause a discharge.

5.39 A. False
  B. True
  C. False
  D. True
  E. True

The exact aetiology of cyclical breast pain is unclear. There are few effective means of treating the condition in all cases. The main aim of the surgeon is to exclude an underlying abnormality. Gammalinoleic acid (evening primrose oil) is helpful in 40–60% of cases. Other drug treatments include danazol, bromocriptine, goserelin and tamoxifen, although the latter is not licensed for use in these cases. Surgery is rarely indicated or helpful.

5.40 A. True
   B. True
   C. False
   D. True
   E. True

Physiological gynaecomastia of puberty is the most common cause in young adults. Other causes include: lung, adrenal and testicular tumour, liver disease, renal failure and hyperprolactinaemia. Drugs also include cimetidine, metoclopramide and tricyclic antidepressants.

5.41 A. False
   B. False
   C. False
   D. False
   E. True

Tamoxifen blocks oestrogen receptors, stimulation of which normally enhances tumour growth. A dose of 20 mg/day improves overall survival and time to recurrence, in both oestrogen positive and oestrogen negative tumours, although the effect is less marked in the second group. Side effects include hot flushes and vaginal dryness, with a small increased risk of endometrial cancer after prolonged treatment. It reduces the risk of associated cardiovascular disease.

5.42 A. True
   B. False
   C. False
   D. False
   E. False

Mutation or loss of heterozygosity of the p53 (tumour suppressor gene) occurs in Li–Fraumeni syndrome. Lynch II syndrome, caused by an autosomal dominant mutation, is also associated with a high risk of breast and ovarian cancer.

5.43 A. True
   B. False
   C. True
   D. True
   E. True

Prolonged exposure to oestrogenic stimulus is a major risk factor for breast cancer. This can happen in nulliparous women with early menarche and late menopause, who may also have had prolonged use of the oral contraceptive pill and hormone replacement therapy. Chest wall irradition, such as in patients with a history of childhood tuberculosis, increases risk. Obesity also shows increased risk, possibly as a result of hormone secretion from fat cells.

5.44 A. False
   B. True
   C. True
   D. False
   E. True

In the TNM classification, T3 is defined by a tumour of greater than 5 cm in any dimension. T4 occurs with skin changes, ulceration or chest wall involvement regardless of size. Fixity of nodes or presence of metastatic disease automatically defines this as advanced breast disease.

5.45 A. False
   B. False
   C. False
   D. True
   E. False

FNA is part of the triple assessment of breast lesions, and is also widely used for other solid lesions. C1 is non-diagnostic. C2 is definitively benign and C5 definitively malignant. It has a very high sensitivity and specificity for diagnosis (> 95%).

5.46 A. False
  B. True
  C. False
  D. True
  E. False

High grade (grade III), ductal-type carcinoma and evidence of vascular invasion all have a poorer prognosis. Expression of the Ki 67 antigen by proliferating cells and large numbers of actively mitotic cells are related to poor prognosis. Expression of hormone receptors is a more favourable prognostic indicator. Other cell wall and gene factors have been implicated as prognostic indices.

5.47 A. False
  B. True
  C. True
  D. False
  E. True

Breast conservation surgery (that is, not total mastectomy) plus radiotherapy gives equivalent survival rates to mastectomy alone. More women are now also opting for total mastectomy and immediate reconstruction.

5.48 A. True
  B. True
  C. False
  D. False
  E. False

Radiotherapy to the axilla is usually contraindicated after axillary level III clearance because of unacceptably high rates of upper limb lymphoedema. The axillary vein marks the upper limit of dissection. The long thoracic nerve, thoracodorsal bundle and pectoralis minor and major muscles are all preserved. Axillary dissection is only indicated in the presence of invasive breast cancer.

5.49 A. False
    B. True
    C. True
    D. False
    E. False

Breast cancer can metastasize haematogenously to bone, lungs, brain, liver and peritoneum with regional symptoms. It has a predilection for bone, with resulting pain, pathological fractures and hypercalcaemia as a result of bone lysis. The mean survival rate is 18–24 months with metastatic disease and the primary aim is to palliate symptoms.

5.50 A. True
    B. False
    C. False
    D. True
    E. False

DCIS may represent preinvasive carcinoma although the exact nature is unclear. There is abnormal proliferation of epithelial cells, but no penetration of the basement membrane. It is often an incidental finding on screening mammography with atypical micro-calcification patterns, and may be multi-focal. It can occur in association with Paget's disease of the nipple.

5.51 A. True
    B. False
    C. False
    D. False
    E. True

Fibroadenomas are the common breast lesions in women under 35 years of age. Diagnosis is, as for any new breast lump, through triple assessment. A proportion will resolve spontaneously, others require excision because of discomfort or patient anxiety. Malignant transformation is very rare.

5.52 A. False
    B. True
    C. True
    D. True
    E. True

Mammary dysplasia covers structural changes in the breast which occur as a result of the physiological responses in puberty (fibroadenoma, single duct obstruction), cyclical change (mastalgia, nodularity), pregnancy (galactocoele), lactation and menopause (sclerosis, adenosis and duct ectasia). The spectrum of change is classified under Aberrations of Normal Development and Involution (ANDI).

5.53 A. True
    B. False
    C. False
    D. True
    E. False

Male breast cancer accounts for 0.5–1% of all breast cancers. It tends to develop in an older population than in women. The main risk factor is hereditary, although there is an association with certain occupations and in patients who are treated with oestrogens for prostatic cancer. The majority of tumours do express hormone receptors and all histological types of tumours are seen. Presentation is usually at a more advanced stage and so overall prognosis is poorer.

5.54 A. False
    B. False
    C. False
    D. True
    E. True

Breast screening is by invitation and therefore overall results vary between regions and socioeconomic classes. The UK screening programme was established in 1988. The hope was that over 70% of women would accept the invitation, and that the death rate would fall by 25%. The results of this initiative still remain under evaluation.

5.55 A. True
   B. True
   C. True
   D. False
   E. True

Bone scans, chest X-rays and liver function tests, with a possible ultrasound scan, aim at excluding the presence of metastatic disease from the most common sites such as bone, lung and liver. A CT of the head is not routinely carried out.

5.56 A. True
   B. False
   C. True
   D. False
   E. False

Regular examination and annual mammography are the mainstay of monitoring breast disease. Bone scans are indicated only if there is a clinical suspicion. CA 153 is a research tumour marker which is often elevated in breast cancer. CEA is a similar research marker in colorectal disease.

5.57 A. False
   B. True
   C. True
   D. True
   E. False

Chemotherapy may be administered as either adjuvant treatment with surgery or as primary treatment in metastatic disease. In the former group, greatest benefit is seen in young patients (premenopausal) with lymph node involvement. There are many side effects including hair loss, nausea and vomiting.

5.58 A. False
  B. True
  C. True
  D. True
  E. False

The latissimus dorsi flap is the most common form of reconstruction offered post breast surgery. The latissimus dorsi muscle and overlying skin are mobilized, and rotated from posterior to anterior on the thoracodorsal pedicle. The skin closes the defect post mastectomy, and the muscle provides bulk, which can be further augmented using a prosthesis or tissue expander.

5.59 A. False
  B. False
  C. False
  D. False
  E. True

A phylloides tumour (cystosarcoma phylloides) can resemble sarcoma histologically, and can behave either as a benign lesion (over 80%) or as an invasive lesion. The size is also variable, but lymph node spread is rare. These tumours are not usually radiosensitive. They occur most commonly among those aged 40–50.

5.60 A. True
  B. False
  C. False
  D. False
  E. False

Clinically, Paget's disease can resemble eczema of the nipple, but is unilateral. It presents as an inflamed or ulcerated lesion, and may indicate an underlying intraduct carcinoma.

5.61 A. False
   B. True
   C. False
   D. False
   E. True

In the TNM classification with regards to breast cancer, T3 relates to tumours over 5 cm. T4 is any size tumour but with skin or chest wall involvement, as in *peau d'orange*. MX implies that the presence of metastasis cannot be determined. N2 indicates fixed homolateral axillary nodes.

5.62 A. True
   B. False
   C. True
   D. True
   E. True

Ductal carcinoma accounts for 90% of cases. Lobular is the next most common, and this is often multicentric and bilateral in 20% of cases. Tubular lesions are usually small and well differentiated. Mucinous tumours are also slow growing and therefore have a better prognosis. They occur in the elderly and the cells lie within pools of mucin. Medullary tumours are characterized by lymphocytic infiltration.

5.63 A. True
   B. True
   C. True
   D. True
   E. False

Fat necrosis occurs after local trauma. It often presents as a hard irregular lump and can easily be mistaken for a carcinoma. Diagnosis is as for any suspicious lump. The condition is self limiting and usually improves spontaneously.

5.64 A. True
    B. False
    C. False
    D. True
    E. True

The BRCA 1 gene is located on the long arm of chromosome 17, and is implicated in approximately 4% of breast cancers. Mutation of this gene increases the lifetime risk of breast cancer, particularly in the premenopausal population. BRCA 2, a second breast cancer gene, has been found on the long arm of chromosome 13. Mutations can be inherited or sporadic. Li–Fraumeni syndrome relates to the p53 suppressor gene.

5.65 A. False
    B. True
    C. False
    D. False
    E. True

Breast cancer is more common in the Western world, and numbers are particularly high among Jewish women of whom the Ashkenazi group show a higher incidence.

5.66 **1.** H
 2. B
 3. E
 4. C
 5. A
 6. A
 7. F
 8. D

The management of breast cancer, as with all malignancies, aims at being either curative or palliative. In elderly patients or those with other medical risk factors, in whom prolongation of life expectancy is not feasible or surgery too risky, hormonal manipulation is the first choice. For women with confirmed breast cancer, the primary course of treatment is surgery plus some form of adjuvant therapy. Surgery is either a form of wide local excision (breast-conserving surgery) plus radiotherapy, or mastectomy (with or without reconstruction). Axillary dissection is at present necessary for all cases of invasive carcinoma, but not in DCIS. Adjuvant treatment with chemotherapy may be given prior to surgery in premenopausal women to 'downgrade' the lesion with regard to size. In most post-menopausal women tamoxifen is given as adjuvant hormonal treatment.

TECHNIQUES AND OUTCOME OF SURGERY

5.67 A. False
 B. True
 C. True
 D. True
 E. True

Consent can be a signed document or given verbally, but must be clearly recorded in the notes. When obtaining an informed consent for surgical procedures, the surgeon should explain details of the condition and prognosis of the proposed treatment. It should include the common and uncommon complications, including the anaesthetic side effects, and alternative treatments should be mentioned. The patient has the right to withdraw consent to treatment at any time.

5.68 A. True
 B. False
 C. True
 D. False

Treatment of patients without their consent does constitute assault and battery by the surgeon. Patients do not have to be told of all the possible outcomes of surgical procedures when obtaining consent. The parents or guardians of minors under the age of 16 should give consent for surgical procedures. The Bolam principle states that a surgeon would not be deemed negligent if his actions were accepted by a responsible body of medical opinion.

5.69 A. False
   B. True
   C. True
   D. False
   E. False

Nausea and vomiting should be treated and there are many antiemetics to choose from. Dry mouth may be caused by opiates. Hyoscine is an antimuscarinic drug and is used to dry up bronchial and salivary secretions. Constipation is usually well relieved by both stimulant and osmotic laxatives. Midazolam is the sedative of choice for use as an antiepileptic and sedative via syringe driver.

5.70 A. False
   B. False
   C. False
   D. True
   E. False

5.71 A. True
   B. False
   C. True
   D. True
   E. True

In palliative care, NSAIDs are useful as analgesics and may be used in combination with other classes of pain killer. There is no maximum dose for morphine: the dose should be titrated to the patient's needs. Diamorphine can be administered via oral, subcutaneous, intramuscular and intravenous routes. Modified-release morphine preparations may be administered once daily. Transdermal patches are effective in delivering analgesic drugs. Opioids may cause nausea, vomiting, constipation and dry mouth. Carbamazepine can help to reduce nerve pain. Corticosteroids can reduce pain by reducing tumour oedema and swelling.

5.72 A. True
   B. False
   C. True
   D. False
   E. False

Nerve blocks can be useful for pain in a region supplied by specific nerves. Transcutaneous electrical nerve stimulation (TENS) may be useful for pain relief. Diazepam can reduce muscle spasm and thus muscle pain. Syringe drivers are used to deliver drugs – for example, analgesics, antiemetics and sedatives – subcutaneously, not intramuscularly.

5.73 A. True
   B. True
   C. True
   D. True
   E. True

Structure, process and outcome are the main types of audit. Structure relates to resources such as manpower and infrastructure. Process relates to all aspects of patient care, from the first moment of contact with the health provider, to discharge from care including treatment. It measures the ability of the system to deliver the healthcare needs of the population.

5.74 A. True
   B. True
   C. True
   D. True
   E. True
   F. True

Outcome audit assesses the results of treatment, all aspects of which are evaluated. This includes morbidity and side effects, mortality, symptom relief, patient satisfaction, quality of life, length of hospital stay and safety.

5.75 A. True
    B. True
    C. False
    D. True
    E. True

Clinical audit is defined by the Department of Health as the systematic, critical analysis of the quality of medical care, including the procedures used for diagnosis and treatment, the use of resources, and the resulting outcome and quality of life for the patient. The audit cycle/loop consists of:
1. Observation of current practice;
2. Setting a standard;
3. Comparison of observed practice with the standard;
4. Implementation of change if required;
5. Comparison of results of new practice with old and an assessment of whether there has been improvement.

5.76 A. False
    B. False
    C. True
    D. True
    E. True

Research seeks to define best practice and determines what constitutes good care. Audit determines if good care is being practised. Clinical trials compare the effect and value of intervention against controls. Clinical audit assesses the total care of the patient by all healthcare professionals, whereas medical audit is assessment of patient care provided by doctors.

Index

A

Abbreviated Injury Scale, 3.20
Abdominal surgery
  incisional hernia, 1.43
  morbid obesity and, 1.21, 2.14
  pleural effusion following, 1.42
  risk assessment, 1.53
  wound dehiscence, 1.10
Abdominal trauma, 3.9–11, 3.35
  penetrating, 3.11, 3.26
Abdominal ultrasound, 2.30
Abscesses
  cerebral, 2.32
  hepatic, 1.15
  paracolic diverticular, 1.15
  superficial, 2.8
Acid—base balance, 4.48
Acidosis
  metabolic, see Metabolic acidosis
  respiratory, cardiopulmonary
    resuscitation and, 4.43
Adenomas, 5.7
Adrenaline, 4.51
  with local anaesthetic, 1.39
Adult respiratory distress syndrome,
    4.29
AIDS, see HIV disease/AIDS
Airway management, 3.2, 3.27, 3.34
Alkalosis
  metabolic, see Metabolic alkalosis
  respiratory, pain causing, 4.48
Alpha-fetoprotein, 5.29
Alveolar partial pressure of oxygen,
    4.6
American Society of
    Anesthesiologists status, 1.53
Anaesthetic, local, see Local
    anaesthetic
Analgesia, 1.35–6
  in palliative care, 5.70–1
  postoperative, 1.35
    haemorroidectomy, 1.49
Angiomyolipoma, 5.31
Antibiotics, 4.21
  prophylactic, 1.10–11, 1.16, 1.31
    colorectal surgery, 1.41, 2.7
    resistance problems, 1.9
  S. aureus sensitivity, 1.45, 2.21

  therapeutic, 1.8
    ascending cholangitis, 1.40
Anticoagulation, 1.19
APACHE II, 3.20
  preoperative, 1.12
Argon laser, 1.50
Arterial blood gases, 2.30
Arterial line in radial artery, 4.35
Arterial partial pressure of oxygen,
    4.6
ASA status, 1.53
Assessment, preoperative, see
    Preoperative assessment
Atrial fibrillation, 4.49
Audit, 5.73–6
Avascular necrosis, 3.33
Axillary nodes, see Lymph nodes

B

Basal metabolic rate, 4.46
Biliary stone, see Gallstones
Biliary stricture, biopsy, 2.33
Biopsy, 2.33
  fine needle aspiration, see Fine
    needle aspiration
Bipolar diathermy, 1.17
Blood, faecal occult, 5.12
Blood flow, cerebral, see Cerebral
    blood flow
Blood gases, arterial, 2.30
Blood loss, trauma patient, 3.3
Blood pressure, see Hypertension;
    Hypotension
Blood transfusion, 1.13, 4.5
Blow-out fracture, 3.25
Blunt trauma
  abdomen, 3.9
  chest, 4.50
Body plethysmography, 4.9
Bone fracture healing, tubular, 1.24
Bone metastases, 5.33
Bowel/intestine
  hamartomatous polyps, 5.5
  obstruction, prolonged, 4.30
  surgery
    anastomosis leak, 2.25
    large bowel, see Colorectal
      surgery

Bowel/intestine (cont'd)
tumours/cancer
large bowel, 1.41, 5.3, 5.12, 5.25, 5.29, 5.33
small bowel, 5.20
Brain abscess, 2.32
Brain death diagnosis, 4.27
BRCA 1 gene, 5.64
Breast, 5.34–65
abscess, 2.8
benign tumours, 5.51, 5.59
enlargement in males, 5.40
fat necrosis, 5.63
fine needle aspiration, 2.33, 5.45
malignant tumours/cancer, 5.39, 5.42–9, 5.53–8, 5.61–2, 5.64–5
axillary clearance/dissection, 5.35, 5.48
carcinoma in situ, ductal, 5.50
chemotherapy, 5.57
conservation surgery, 5.47
first-line management, 5.66
genetics, 5.64
hormone therapy, 5.28, 5.41
locally advanced, 5.44
males, 5.53
metastases, 5.33, 5.49, 5.55
mortalities, 5.1
mucinous carcinoma, 5.62
newly-diagnosed, staging, 5.55
palliative therapy, 5.33
post-treatment follow-up, 5.56
prognosis, 5.15, 5.46
risk factors/epidemiology, 5.42–3, 5.65
screening, 5.54
TNM staging, 5.32, 5.44, 5.60
tumour markers, 5.15
types, 5.62
mammography, 5.37
pain, cyclical, 5.39
reconstruction, 5.58
Bronchospasm, 4.45
Brush cytology, 2.33
Bullet wound, see Missile wound
Burns, 3.23

C
CA 125, 5.29
CA 153, 5.15
CA 19–9, 5.29
Calcium disturbances, post-thyroidectomy, 4.42
Campylobacter spp., 2.31
Cancer, see Tumours
Carbon dioxide laser, 1.50
Carbon monoxide poisoning, 4.17

Carcinoembryonic antigen, 5.29
Carcinogens, physical/chemical, 5.30
Carcinoid tumours, 5.15
Cardiac drugs, 4.51
Cardiac failure
drug therapy, 4.51
intra-aortic balloon pumps, 4.24
Cardiac tamponade, 3.8
Cardiopulmonary resuscitation, 4.43
Central venous pressure elevation and hypotension, 4.31
Cerebral abscess, 2.32
Cerebral blood flow, 4.24
autoregulation, 3.13, 4.24
Cerebral perfusion pressure, 3.13
Cerebrospinal fluid, 3.14
Cervical dermatomes, 3.18
Cervical spinal cord injury, 3.19
in unconscious patient, signs, 4.36
Chemotherapy, 5.25–7
breast cancer, 5.57, 5.66
Chest
flail, 3.5, 3.6, 3.7
injuries, 3.5–8, 3.36, 4.50
Chest drains, 3.7, 3.36
Chest X-ray, 1.18, 2.2, 4.1
Chief Triage Officer, 3.27
Cholangitis, ascending, 1.40
Choledocholithiasis, see Gallstones
Choriocarcinoma, 5.27
Clostridia spp., 1.14
botulinum, 2.31
tetani (and tetanus), 1.29–30, 4.19
Coagulation, disseminated intravascular, 4.37
Colorectal surgery, 2.24, see also Bowel
antibiotic prophylaxis, 2.7
Colorectal tumours/cancer, 1.41, 5.3, 5.12, 5.25, 5.29, 5.33
Compartment syndrome, 3.33
Computed tomography, abdominal trauma, 3.10, 3.11, 3.35
Consent, informed, 5.67–8
Continuous mandatory ventilation, 4.10
Continuous positive airways pressure, 4.10
Core needle biopsy, 2.33
Cranium, see Skull
Cricothyroidotomy, 3.34
Curtis—Fitz—Hugh syndrome, 1.15
Cushing's reflex, 3.13
Cyproterone acetate, 5.28
Cystosarcoma phylloides, 5.59
Cytotoxic anticancer drugs, see Chemotherapy

D

Deep vein thrombosis, see Venous thrombosis
Dehiscence, abdominal wound, 1.10
Dermatomes, cervical, 3.18
Diabetes
  ASA status, 1.53
  ECG, preoperative, 2.5
  insulin-dependent, 2.1
Diamorphine, 5.70, 5.71, 5.72
Diaphragmatic rupture, 3.5, 3.6, 3.7
Diaphyseal/tubular bone fracture healing, 1.24, 3.31
Diathermy
  bipolar, 1.17
  monopolar, 2.10
Diclofenac, 1.36
Disseminated intravascular coagulation, 4.37
Dobutamine, 4.50, 4.51
Dopamine, intravenous, 4.11
Drains
  chest, 3.7, 3.36
  T-tube, 2.26
Ductal carcinoma, 5.62
Ductal carcinoma in situ, 5.50
Dysplasia, mammary, 5.52

E

ECG, see Electrocardiogram
Electrocardiogram (ECG), 4.3, 4.41
  in hyperkalaemia, 4.23
  preoperative, 2.5
  QRS complex/interval, 4.3, 4.23
  QT interval, 4.23, 4.41
  ST segment depression, 4.23
  T wave, 4.23, 4.41
Electrocautery, 1.17, see also Diathermy
Electrolyte infusion, 4.12, 4.13
Embolism
  cerebral, 4.35
  fat, 3.33, 4.33
  pulmonary, 2.30, 4.35, 4.49
Endocrine therapy, see Hormone therapy
Endoscopic biopsy, 2.33
Endoscopic retrograde cholangiopancreatography, 1.40
Endotracheal intubation, see Intubation
Ephedrine, 4.51
Epiphyseal fractures healing, 3.31
Escherichia coli, 2.31
Extradural haematoma, 3.15, 3.16

F

Faecal occult blood, 5.12
Fat embolism, 3.33, 4.33
Fat necrosis of breast, 5.63
Femoral fractures, 3.33
Femoral nerve, 3.30
Fentanyl, 4.15
Fever, see Pyrexia
Fibroadenomas, 5.51
Fibrocystic disease of breast (=mammary dysplasia), 5.52
Fine needle aspiration (percutaneous), 2.33
  breast, 2.33, 5.45
  lung, 1.25
Flail chest, 3.5, 3.6, 3.7
Flaps, 3.22
  breast reconstruction, 5.58
Fluid resuscitation, 4.13, 4.50
Forced expired volume in 1 second, 4.7
Fractures
  healing, see Healing
  maxillary, 3.24
  orbital blow-out, 3.25
  pelvic, 3.12
  skull, 3.16
Fresh frozen plasma, 2.6
Functional residual capacity, 4.2, 4.7, 4.9

G

Gallstones (choledocholithiasis), 2.30
  removal, 1.40
Gangrene, synergistic, 1.14
Gas gangrene, 1.14
Gastrectomy, total, 1.20
Gastric cancer, 1.20, 5.1, 5.2
Gastrointestinal lymphoma, 5.20
Glyceryl trinitrate, 4.51
Glycine irrigation, 4.32
Gonadotrophin-releasing hormone analogues, 5.28
Grafts, skin, 3.21
Gunshot wound, see Missile wound
Gynaecomastia, 5.40

H

Haematoma
  intracranial, 3.15, 3.16
  wound, post-thyroidectomy, 4.42
Haemoglobin
  oxygen dissociation curve, 4.39
  oxygen saturation, estimation, 4.8
Haemolytic transfusion reactions, 4.5
Haemorroidectomy, analgesia after, 1.49

Haemothorax, 3.8, 3.36
Hamartomatous polyps, 5.5
Head injury, 3.13, 3.15–17, 3.34
Healing and repair (wound), 1.11
    burns, 3.23
    factors adversely affecting, 1.33
    fracture, 3.31
        delayed union, 3.32
        tubular/diaphyseal bone, 1.24,
            3.31
    by secondary intention, 1.1, 1.10,
        3.28
Heart, see entries under Cardiac
Helium dilution technique, 4.9
Hemicolectomy, right, 2.24
Heparin, 1.19
Hepatocellular carcinoma, 5.29, 5.30
Hepatology, see Liver
Hernia, abdominal incisional, 1.43
HIV disease/AIDS, 1.32
    complications, 1.27
Hodgkin's disease, 5.18
Hormone therapy
    breast cancer, 5.28, 5.41, 5.66
    prostate cancer, 5.28
Hyperkalaemia, 4.24
    ECG, 4.23
Hypertension
    ECG in, 2.5
    surgical risk, 2.13
        assessment, 1.53
Hyperventilation and head injury,
    3.17
Hypocalcaemia, post-thyroidectomy,
    4.42
Hypokalaemia, metabolic alkalosis in,
    4.48
Hyponatraemia, 4.14, 4.32
Hypotension, 1.40, 4.31, 4.49
    central venous pressure elevation
        and, 4.31
    in cervical spinal cord injury,
        3.19
    in head injury, 3.17
    intracranial pressure in, 3.13
    warm/cold, 1.3

I
Immunocompromised persons, 1.32,
    2.23
Incisional hernia, abdominal, 1.43
Infection, 2.31–2, see also Gangrene;
        Osteomyelitis; Sepsis and
        specific pathogens
    perioperative, 1.15–16
        AIDS-related, 1.27
        endogenous, 2.22
        prevention, 1.4, 1.16, 2.16

    risk factor, 1.9
    transfusion-related, 1.13, 4.5
    treatment, 1.7–8
    wound, see Wound
    staff precautions, 2.9
Inflammation, wound, 1.6
Injury, see Trauma
Injury Severity Score, 3.20
Insulin-dependent diabetes, 2.1
Intensive care, 4.1–51
Intercostal space, 5th, thoracotomy,
    2.27
Intermittent positive pressure
    ventilation, 4.10
Intestine, see Bowel
Intra-aortic balloon pumps, 4.24
Intracerebral embolism, 4.35
Intracranial haematoma, 3.15, 3.16
Intracranial pressure, 3.13, 3.44
Intubation, endotracheal, 3.2
    bronchospasm with, 4.45
    head injury, 3.17
        face/maxilla/skull base, 3.24,
            3.34
Investigations, 2.30
Iodine-131, thyroid cancer, 1.22

J
Jaundice, obstructive, 2.15
Juxtaglomerular tumour, 5.31

K
Keloid scars, 1.46, 2.17, 2.18
Kidney
    drugs affecting, 4.20, 4.21
    tumours, 5.13–14, 5.31

L
Laminar flow, 1.4, 1.17
Laparotomy
    blunt trauma, 3.10
    gastric cancer preoperative
        staging, 1.20
    gunshot wound, 3.11
    immediate, 3.35
Laryngeal mask airway, 3.2
Laryngeal stridor, post-
    thyroidectomy, 4.42
Laser surgery, 1.50
    Nd-YAG laser, 1.50, 2.11
Latissimus dorsi flap, 5.58
Le Fort I-III fractures, 3.24
Leukaemia, 5.27
Li-Fraumeni syndrome, 5.42, 5.64 •
Lignocaine, 2.28
Liver
    abscesses, 1.15
    cancer, 5.29, 5.30

secondary, 5.12, 5.33
failure, acute, 4.38
Lobular carcinoma of breast, 5.62
Local anaesthetic, 2.28–9
　with adrenaline, 1.39
Lumbosacral myotomes, 3.18
Lung
　contusions, 3.5, 3.6
　functions, tests, 4.2, 4.7, 4.9
　masses, 1.51
　　fine needle aspiration of lung,
　　　1.25
　volumes, 4.2
Lung cancer/carcinoma, 1.51, 5.10–11
　fine needle aspiration, 1.25
　secondary (from renal cell cancer),
　　5.14
　tumour markers, 5.15
Lymph nodes, axillary (in breast
　　cancer)
　clearance/dissection, 5.35, 5.48,
　　5.66
　in TNM staging, 5.32, 5.44, 5.60
Lymphoblastic leukaemia, acute, 5.27
Lymphoma, 5.18–20
　gastrointestinal, 5.20
　Hodgkin's, 5.18
　non-Hodgkin's, 5.19
Lynch II syndrome, 5.42

M
Magnetic resonance imaging, 2.3
Major incidents, 3.27
Malignant tumours, see Tumours
Mammary dysplasia, 5.52
Mammography, breast, 5.37
Mannitol, 4.44
Mastalgia, cyclical, 5.39
Mastectomy, 5.66
Maxillary fractures, 3.24
　intubation, 3.24, 3.34
Median nerve, 3.29
Mediastinal traversing wounds, 3.7
Medullary carcinoma of breast, 5.62
Melanoma, malignant, 5.17
　biopsy, 2.33
　characteristics, 5.17
　chemotherapy, 5.27
　risk factors, 5.4, 5.17
Meleney's burrowing ulcer, 1.14
Mesothelioma, 5.30
Metabolic acidosis, 1.2, 4.26
　cardiopulmonary resuscitation and,
　　4.43
Metabolic alkalosis, 4.34
　in hypokalaemia, 4.48
Metastases, see also TNM staging
　bone, 5.33

liver, 5.12, 5.33
origin
　breast cancer, 5.33 5.49, 5.55
　colorectal cancer, 5.12, 5.25
　renal cell cancer, 5.13
process of metastasis, 5.8
Methicillin-resistant *S. aureus*, 1.45,
　　2.21
Methylprednisolone in spinal cord
　　injury, 4.18
Midazolam, 4.15
Minor surgery, 2.17
Missile (gunshot/bullet) wound, 3.26
　abdominal, 3.11, 3.26
　chest, 3.36
Mitozantrone, 5.25
Monopolar diathermy, 2.10
Morphine
　bronchospasm with, 4.45
　in palliative care, 5.70, 5.71
　as sedative, 4.15
Multiple injuries, 3.35
　airway management, 3.2
　initial assessment, 3.1
Musculocutaneous nerve, 3.29
Myocutaneous flaps, 3.22
Myotomes, lumbosacral, 3.18

N
Naloxone, 4.47
Nasal cavity cancer, 5.30
Nasopharyngeal airway, 3.2
Nasotracheal intubation and
　　maxillofacial fracture, 3.24,
　　3.34
Necrotizing fasciitis, 1.5, 2.32
Neodymium-YAG laser, 1.50, 2.11
Neoplasia, see Tumours
Nerves, 3.29–30
　injury, 3.30
　　in minor surgery, 2.17
Neuron-specific enolase, 5.15
Nipple
　discharge, 5.38
　Paget's disease, 5.60
Nitrogen washout technique, 4.9
Nitroglycerin (GTN), 4.51
Non-Hodgkin's lymphoma, 5.19
Non-steroidal anti-inflammatory
　　drugs (NSAIDs), 1.36, 5.71
Noradrenaline, 4.51
Nutritional replacement, 4.13

O
Oat cell (small cell) carcinoma of
　　lung, 5.11, 5.16
Obesity, morbid, 1.23
　abdominal surgery and, 1.21, 2.14

Occipital lobes, 3.14
Oculomotor nerve compression, 3.14
Oestrogens and breast cancer, 5.43
Oliguria, 4.50
Oncogenes, 5.16
Opioids
    antagonists, 4.47
    bronchospasm with, 4.45
    in palliative care, 5.70, 5.71, 5.72
    postoperative, 1.35
    as sedatives, 4.15
Orbital blow-out fracture, 3.25
Oropharyngeal airway, 3.2
Orotracheal intubation, 3.34
    maxillofacial fracture, 3.24, 3.34
Orthopantomogram, 3.24
Osteogenic sarcoma, 5.27
Osteomyelitis, acute, 1.26
Osteoporotic fractures, 3.32
Ovarian cancer, 5.29
Oximetry, pulse, 3.1, 4.8
Oxygen
    alveolar partial pressure of, 4.6
    arterial partial pressure of, 4.6
    haemoglobin saturation,
        estimation, 4.8
Oxyhaemoglobin dissociation curve,
    4.39

P
p53 gene, 5.16
Pacemakers and monopolar
    diathermy, 2.10
Paget's disease of nipple, 5.60
Pain
    breast, cyclical, 5.39
    relief, see Analgesia
    visceral, 1.37–8
Palliative care, 5.33, 5.69–72
Pancreatic cancer, 5.1, 5.27, 5.29, 5.33
Pancreatitis, 1.15
Paracolic diverticular abscesses, 1.15
Paralysis
    in spinal cord injury, 3.19
    ventilation in, 4.10
Pelvic fractures, 3.12
Penetrating abdominal trauma, 3.11,
    3.26, 3.35
Percutaneous fine needle aspiration
    of lung, 1.25
Perianal abscess, 2.8
Peritoneal lavage, diagnostic, 3.9,
    3.10, 3.11, 3.12, 3.35
Peritonitis, 1.15, 2.26
Peroneal nerve injury
    common, 3.30
    superficial, 3.30
Pethidine, 4.15, 4.45

Peutz—Jeghers syndrome, 5.5
Photodynamic laser, 1.50
Phylloides tumour, 5.59
Plethysmography, body, 4.9
Pleural effusion, post-abdominal
    surgery, 1.42
Pneumonia, 1.51
Pneumothorax, 3.36
    open, 3.5, 3.6, 3.7
    tension, 3.4, 3.5, 3.6, 4.49
Polyps, hamartomatous, 5.5
Positive end-expiratory pressure, 4.10
Posterior cranial fossa, 3.14
Potassium
    disturbances, see Hyperkalaemia;
        Hypokalaemia
    replacement, 4.13
PR interval, 4.3, 4.41
Precentral gyrus, 3.14
Preoperative assessment
    APACHE II system, 1.12
    of surgical risk, 1.53
Pressure support ventilation, 4.10
Primary Triage Officer, 3.27
Prostate cancer, 5.28, 5.29
Prostate-specific antigen, 5.29
Pulmonary artery floatation catheter,
    4.4
Pulmonary embolism, 2.30, 4.35, 4.49
Pulmonary non-vascular tissue, see
    Lung
Pulse oximetry, 3.1, 4.8
Pupillary signs, 3.14, 3.17
Pyrexia (fever), postoperative, 1.44
    post-bowel surgery, 2.25
    post-ERCP, 1.40

R
Radial artery, arterial line, 4.35
Radial nerve, 3.29
Radiograph, see X-ray
Radiotherapy, 5.21–4
    axillary node, 5.48
    palliative, 5.33
Rectum
    antibiotic prophylaxis for surgery,
        1.41, 2.7
    cancer, 1.41, 5.3, 5.12, 5.29, 5.33
    injury, 3.12
Rectus abdominis myocutaneous
    flap, transverse, 3.22
Renal cell cancer, 5.13–14, 5.31
Renal problems, see Kidney
Respiratory acidosis,
    cardiopulmonary resuscitation
        and, 4.43
Respiratory alkalosis, pain causing,
    4.48

Respiratory distress syndrome, adult,
    4.29
Respiratory tract infection,
    community-acquired, 2.32
Retinoblastoma gene, 5.16
Revised Trauma Score, 3.20
Rhabdomyolysis, 4.28

S
Salicylate poisoning, 4.16
Sarcoma, osteogenic, 5.27
Scaphoid fractures, 3.33
Scars, keloid, 1.46, 2.17, 2.18
Sciatic nerve, 3.30
Sedation, 4.15
Sepsis, 4.49, 4.51
    postoperative, 1.44, 2.20
        shock due to, 1.3
Shock
    septic, 1.3
    in trauma, 3.1, 3.3
Sickle cell testing, 2.4
Skin
    biopsy, 2.33
    malignancy, see Melanoma
Skin grafts, 3.21
Skull/cranium
    fracture, 3.16
    gunshot wounds, 3.26
    posterior fossa, 3.14
    X-ray, 3.17, 3.24
Small bowel
    hamartomatous polyps, 5.5
    lymphoma, 5.20
Small cell carcinoma of lung, 5.11,
    5.16
Sodium
    disturbances, 4.14, 4.32
    replacement, 4.13
Spinal cord, 3.18
    injury, 3.19, 4.18
        in unconscious patient, signs,
        4.36
Spinothalamic tract, 3.18
Spirometry, 4.7
Staphylococci spp., 1.5, 1.14
    aureus, antibiotic sensitivity, 1.45,
    2.21
Sterilization (instruments), 1.52
Stomach, see entries under Gastr-
Stones, biliary, see Gallstones
Streptococci spp., 1.5, 1.14
    milleri, 2.32
    pneumoniae, 2.32
    pyogenes, 2.32
Subdural haematoma, 3.16
Suturing, 1.10, 1.17
Synchronized positive pressure

ventilation, 4.10
Systemic immune response
    syndrome, 1.3

T
T-tube drains, 2.26
Talar fractures, 3.33
Tamoxifen, 5.28, 5.41, 5.66
Tension pneumothorax, 3.4, 3.5, 3.6,
    4.49
Tetanus, 1.29–30, 4.19
Thoracotomy, 2.27
    resuscitative/immediate, 3.8
Thrombocytopenia, 2.12
Thyroid cancer, 1.22, 5.30
Thyroidectomy, 4.42
Thyroxine, thyroid cancer, 1.22
Tibial nerve, 3.30
TNM staging, breast cancer, 5.32,
    5.44, 5.61
Tracheal intubation, see Intubation
Tracheostomy, 1.47
Transurethral resection syndrome,
    4.32
Transverse rectus abdominis
    myocutaneous flap, 3.22
Trauma, 3.1–36
    body's response, 1.34
    minor surgery-related, 2.17
    multiple, see Multiple injuries
    scoring systems, 3.20
    spinal cord, 3.19, 4.14
Triage, 3.27
TRISS, 3.20
Tuberculosis, 1.51
Tubular carcinoma of breast, 5.62
Tumour(s) (predominantly malignant
        = cancer), 5.1–33
    benign vs malignant, 5.6, 5.9
    breast, see Breast
    chemical/physical agents causing,
    5.30
    chemotherapy, see Chemotherapy
    colorectal, 1.41, 5.3, 5.12, 5.25,
    5.29, 5.33
    gastric, 1.20, 5.1, 5.2
    liver, see Liver
    lung, see Lung cancer
    molecular basis of cancer, 5.8, 5.16
    mortalities, 5.1
    nasal cavity, 5.30
    ovarian, 5.29
    pancreatic, 5.1, 5.27, 5.29, 5.33
    prostate, 5.28, 5.29
    radiotherapy, see Radiotherapy
    renal, 5.13–14, 5.31
    secondary, see Metastases
    small bowel, 5.20

Tumour(s) (cont'd)
   thyroid, 1.22, 5.30
   urinary tract, 5.30
   uterine, 5.1
Tumour markers, 5.15, 5.29
Tumour suppressor genes, 5.16

U
Ulnar nerve, 3.29
Ultrasound, abdominal, 2.30
Urinary tract cancer, 5.30
Urine output, 4.50
Uterine cancer mortalities, 5.1

V
Vancomycin, 4.21
Venous thrombosis, deep
   diagnosis, 1.48
   risk factors, 1.28, 4.18
Ventilation (operating room),
   1.4
Ventilation (patient), mechanical, in
   paralysis, 4.10
Ventilation/perfusion ratio, low, 4.6
Vincristine, 5.25, 5.26

Visceral injury, 3.11, 3.12
Visceral pain, 1.37–8
Vital capacity, 4.2
Vomiting, 4.40

W
Wound, surgical
   abdominal, dehiscence, 1.10
   haematoma, post-thyroidectomy,
      4.42
   healing/repair, see Healing
   infection, 1.45
      characteristics, 1.6
      management, 1.7
      in minor surgery, 2.17
      prevention, 2.16
   inflammation, 1.6
Wound, traumatic, management,
   3.28

X
X-ray
   breast, 5.37
   chest, 1.18, 2.2, 4.1
   head/skull, injury, 3.17, 3.24